Cry of the Eagle
By: David Young, Grant Ingram,
Lise Swartz

Cry of the Eagle

Encounters with a Cree Healer

DAVID YOUNG

GRANT INGRAM

LISE SWARTZ

University of Toronto Press
Toronto Buffalo London

© University of Toronto Press Incorporated 1989
Toronto Buffalo London
Printed in Canada
Reprinted in paperback, 1990, 1992, 1997

ISBN 0-8020-6820-0

Printed on acid-free paper

Canadian Cataloguing in Publication Data

Young, David E.
  Cry of the eagle

  Bibliography: p.
  Includes index.
  ISBN 0-8020-6820-0

  1. Willier, Russell.   2. Indians of North America – Canada, Northern –
Medicine.   3. Cree Indians – Medicine.   4. Indians of North America –
Canada, Northern – Biography.   5. Cree Indians – Biography.   6. Shamans
– Alberta – Biography.   I. Ingram, Grant.   II. Swartz, Lise, 1944–
III. Title.

E99.C88W54   1989   971.2'00497   C89-094258-7

This book has been published with the assistance of the Canada Council
and the Ontario Arts Council under their block grant programs.

❦ Contents

❧ Preface

This book is an account of the world as seen through the eyes of Russell Willier, a Woods Cree medicine man from northern Alberta whose medicine name is Mehkwasskwan or Red Cloud. The preceding statement needs to be qualified, however, because the book has been written by anthropologists who are well aware of the fact that no one can see reality through someone else's eyes. Even if Russell Willier had written the book himself, much of the reality of his inner vision would have been lost because of the limitations of the written word. We should say, therefore, that this book is an account of what a Cree medicine man was able to express to outsiders about the way he perceives the world and how he attempts to transform his vision into action.

It is rare for medicine men to provide in-depth information to outsiders. The authors' relationship with Russell Willier began by accident. David Young, a professor of anthropology at the University of Alberta, and Gertrude Nicks, the curator of ethnology at the Provincial Museum of Alberta, were studying endangered native crafts in northern Alberta. After having documented the making of birch-bark baskets by elderly women on the Assumption Reserve near High Level, they stopped at the vocational training school in Grouard, a small town approximately three hundred kilometres north of Edmonton, Alberta, to see if they could be introduced to someone with expertise in native skin tanning. Mary Periard, director of the native arts and crafts program at the school, called Russell Willier and his wife, Yvonne, on the telephone, as they had both been involved in demonstrating tanning with animal brains. Russell, who lives on the Sucker Creek Reserve near Grouard, consented to talk to Young and Nicks. After about an hour of conversation, he decided they were trustworthy and invited them to his home to watch him and his wife work skins. It was soon arranged that David Young would return for an extended stay. David and two professional photographers spent the next few weeks photographing and videotaping the methods by which moose skins are processed and made into clothing and items such as drums. Young had no idea at the time that Russell was a practising shaman.

As Russell Willier and David Young got to know each other better, Russell began to reveal more and more about his activities as a medicine man. David Young was extremely interested, and before long he and Russell were discussing the possibility of an anthropological study of Russell's life as a medicine man. Russell expressed a wish to have the power of his healing ability documented 'in black and white' in order to prove to the medical establishment that Indian medicine has value and to motivate young natives to have pride in their heritage. David put together a team of researchers at the University of Alberta, and Russell agreed to come to Edmonton to treat psoriasis patients in a downtown health clinic where the results could be observed and documented.

The Psoriasis Research Project led to other kinds of encounters with Russell Willier and, eventually, to this book. The first chapter provides an overview of the actors and setting. Chapters two, three, and four deal with Russell Willier's view of the cosmos. Chapters five, six, and seven describe how Russell translates his view of the world into action. The final chapter illustrates what Russell is doing to help traditional native medicine adapt to non-native society.

Academic writing is frequently dull and irrelevant because the human element is left out. Anthropological theory, moreover, tends to be discussed in the abstract. In this book we provide an intimate glimpse into the life and thought of a real person and embed the theoretical points we wish to make in ethnographic description. Although we hope the book will be of interest to professional anthropologists, we decided to avoid the use of academic references and to write in a style that will be understood easily by the intelligent layperson who has an interest in anthropology. At the end of the book the reader will find a short list of publications that we have consulted or that have influenced our thinking in a significant way. Our own publications are included in the list.

We use three different terms to describe Russell Willier's activities, depending upon the context: 'shaman,' 'medicine man,' and 'healer.' A shaman is mainly concerned with mediating between 'supernatural' powers and humans; a medicine man uses natural substances such as herbs and animal parts and/or spiritual means to effect cures and to repel curses; and a healer treats specific problems using traditional techniques. Although Russell acknowledges the appropriateness of all three terms, he prefers to be called a medicine man. It should be noted that there are also many medicine women.

The book has involved a joint effort in all respects, but each chapter has been the primary responsibility of a single author. David Young wrote chapters one, two, seven, and eight, Grant Ingram chapters three and five, and Lise Swartz chapters four and six. In most cases, we have used fictitious names for the people in the book.

We offer thanks to Russell and Yvonne Willier for sharing their lives and dreams with us and to Joe Cardinal for sharing his knowledge of Grouard in the early days. We also wish to acknowledge the efforts of those who helped with various aspects of the research: Janice Morse, Ruth McConnell, William Ayer, Lois Browne, Kyoko Nishizawa, Joel Wilbush, Alice Hanson, Don Spence, Ken Pappes, Larry Benson, Hari Chana, Hubert Kammerer, Steven Aung, Brian Noble, Judith Golub, Carl Wolgien, and Marna Bunnell. We are grateful to the patients who allowed themselves to be photographed and interviewed and to our families who have been so helpful throughout the past several years. We have appreciated the generous support of the Provincial Museum of Alberta and the following units at the University of Alberta: the Boreal Institute for Northern Studies, the Central Research Fund, the Department of Anthropology, the Faculty of Nursing, and the Department of Radio and Television. We were fortunate in having Leonard Smith, who works with our own Project for the Study of Traditional Healing Practices, as well as Virgil Duff, Margaret Allen, and Lorraine Ourom, of the University of Toronto Press, as our editors.

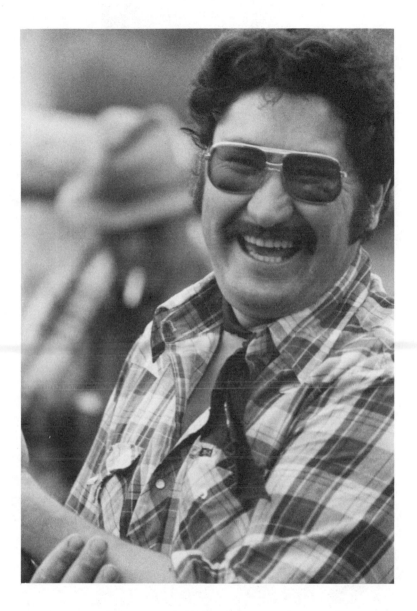

Russell Willier, Woods Cree medicine man, 1983
Courtesy Brian Noble

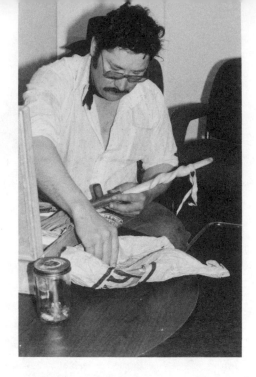

The Psoriasis Research Project: Russell prepares the pipe before treating
patients, 1985.
Courtesy Ruth McConnell, Provincial Museum of Alberta

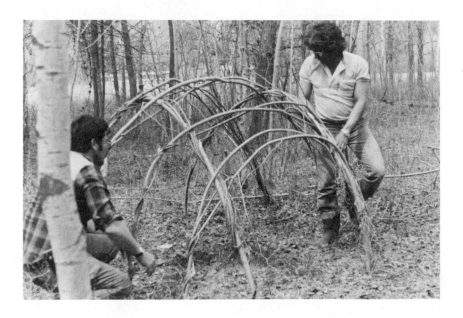

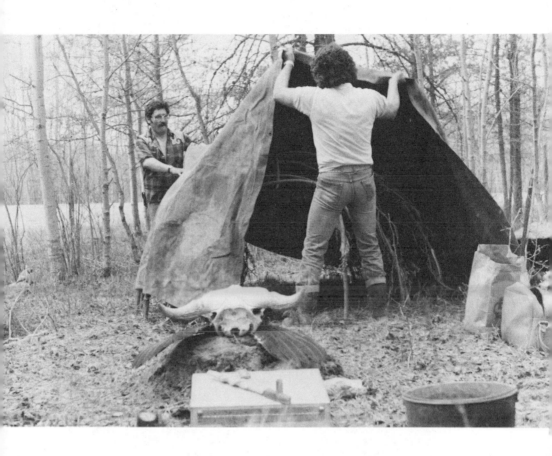

Russell and his nephew drape tarps over the sweat-lodge frame, 1985.
Courtesy David Young

OPPOSITE
Russell and his nephew tie willow saplings to form the roof of the
sweat-lodge, 1985.
Courtesy David Young

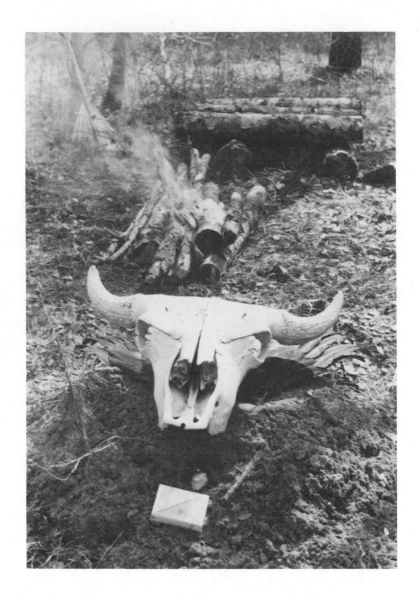

Tobacco offering placed before a buffalo skull and eagle wings on the altar, 1985
Courtesy David Young

CRY OF THE EAGLE

✹ Overview

This book is an attempt to understand our encounter with one man, Russell Willier, a Woods Cree healer, and what he was willing to share with us about himself. In the eyes of many people the world-view of one man, however comprehensive and however eloquently expressed, has little scientific value because one man can't speak for his profession, his community, or his tribe as a whole. Although there is some merit to this argument, frankly we do not know where else to start except with a real person. It's not that we haven't received adequate training as anthropologists. Rather, we have become increasingly convinced that in their attempt to understand the world many social scientists use methods and produce data that have very little to do with reality. We have become tired of reading uninspired treatises about issues that may be important but that could not possibly be understood on the basis of the information collected. Frequently, the need to collect data from large numbers of people means that only very superficial questions can be asked. The resulting generalizations may be well supported, but they are based upon such a thin slice of reality that they run the danger of being trivial.

We prefer the in-depth approach. In a living person reality comes together in a meaningful way. What do we mean by this? One of the primary goals of anthropology is to understand the complex interactions among environment, biology, psychology, and culture. The magnitude of the task means that such understanding is seldom achieved. What better way to begin to pursue this goal than to study a specific individual? It is in an individual that all these variables come together in a living system.

We are not implying that in this book we will be providing information on what happens in Russell Willier's brain or hormonal system as he utilizes cultural information in the pursuit of individual goals. This is beyond the ability of any scientist at the present time. What we can do is to provide information about Russell's understanding of the environment and its potential as a natural medicine cabinet, his understanding of the relationship between physiology and psychology in the maintenance of health and the causation of disease, and his understanding of the interaction between the human and spiritual worlds. The description of Russell Willier's view of the world and of how it works will be supplemented with observations about Russell's activities, the effectiveness of his therapeutic techniques, and the role of his own personality in his medical practice.

Any individual has to take a holistic, ecological perspective if she or he is to cope successfully with a changing environment, whether that environment is a physical or a social one. If we wish anthropology to be holistic and ecological, it makes some sense to regard the world-view and coping strategies of real people as important sources of data. The intent of this book, however, is not to produce a biographical sketch of an interesting individual. It is to see an individual as the focal point of adaptation. Too often, the concept of adaptation (one of the key concepts in anthropology, along with concepts like evolution and culture) is dealt with at such an abstract level that it is almost meaningless. Studying adaptation at the individual level involves attempting to understand how a person puts a great variety of information together in such a way that the world becomes more predictable, meaningful, and congenial to human effort. Anthropological analysis provides information on how this is done by an individual from a specific cultural background and also attempts to shed some light on how this is done by our species as a whole. The ultimate goal is not ethnographic description but insight concerning a fundamental *process*, the process of attempting to move through life in a way that brings the greatest rewards to the individual actor. Viewed from this perspective, an in-depth study of one individual is not as limited in scope as it might first appear.

There will always be a place for highly technical material of interest to a select group of scholars. As professional anthropologists we all engage in what, to outsiders, might look like esoteric research and writing. This is as it should be; yet we have an ethical obligation to share whatever insights we might glean from our research with the world in general. To orient a piece of writing to the general public does not mean that the account must be watered down or devoid of theory. It simply means that theory and description should be integrated into a single whole. All of us tend to forget analytic observations more easily than information about actual events and situations. Theoretical insights embedded in concrete observations are more likely to have an enduring impact.

In this book we have tried to use ordinary language and to portray Russell Willier's view of the world in such a way that some of our own fundamental insights about the mission of the social sciences will also be served. The reader might be tempted to ask: 'Is it fair to pretend to speak for another person while really speaking for yourself?' Although we can't be sure, we think it is fair. We at least are conscious that we are doing what many social scientists do unconsciously. It is impossible to keep personal biases out of research and writing, so why not turn necessity into a virtue? We can serve Russell Willier's and our own interests at the same time, which seems to be an ideal situation and the only way to avoid exploitation.

The question arises as to how Russell Willier believes he can benefit from the co-operative endeavour that led to the writing of this book. Russell Willier has a vision. He is the great-grandson of Moostoos, a noted healer and leader who signed a treaty on behalf of his people with the government many years ago. Like other treaties, Treaty 8 produced some good and some bad results. The reservation system, supposedly a bulwark against the encroachment of 'white' culture, has not always been effective in preserving native ways. On many reserves the traditional ways of healing are in danger of being lost as young people look to the outside world for their models of reality. Tradition is often disparaged, becoming a source of embarrassment to young people. Russell Willier hopes to reverse this trend. He hopes that co-operating with anthropologists will help the world understand that native ways have validity and that native healing techniques are efficacious. If this can be done, young people may be inspired to take pride in their culture and carry on the great healing traditions of the past.

Russell Willier aspires to be a 'cultural broker,' an individual who straddles two cultures for the purpose of creating greater communication and understanding between them. He believes native ways can survive only if native people learn to compete more effectively with non-native institutions, including the health care system. As long as native medicine is kept underground – and regarded as quackery or witch doctoring – it cannot fulfil its proper role in helping Indian people 'stay on the Sweetgrass Trail.' Russell feels that native medicine must come out into the open, demonstrate its effectiveness to both natives and non-natives, and adopt techniques and organizational structures that will earn wide respect. For these reasons, Russell Willier has allowed his healing rituals to be videotaped and photographed. He has also consented to have the results of our research published in scholarly journals and to have his ideas and practices described in this book, which is aimed at a general audience.

Several years ago Russell had a vision. He saw himself in front of a multitude of native people who could not speak for themselves because they had no tongues. As the only one with a tongue, Russell knew that he had been selected to speak on their behalf, to be a leader of a revitalization movement. One of Russell's main spirit helpers, the eagle, which represents far-sightedness and transcendence, symbolizes much of what this vision has come to mean. Inspired by the eagle, Russell envisions natives like himself promoting native ways, not by a return to the old days, but by transcending tradition and moving toward a creative metamorphosis that will strengthen native people's role in society. This is a courageous and controversial vision. Just as the cry of the eagle connotes majesty and danger, Russell's vision of the future inspires awe and fear. It is earning Russell both friends and enemies.

THE ACTORS

It has been common in recent years for social scientists to use metaphors derived from drama and the theatre to describe what they study. This is appropriate in our case; the beliefs and events outlined in this book *are* dramatic. Russell Willier views the world as a battleground for cosmic forces of good and evil, a world in which nothing happens by chance and where great emphasis is put upon divining the future and beseeching spiritual forces for help. The term 'actor' is appropriate in that the encounter between ourselves and Russell required us all to play roles that were in many ways unfamiliar to us. All of us used some well-rehearsed lines from our own cultural settings and backgrounds, but we also did a lot of ad-libbing. The main actors are Russell Willier and the authors of this book, David Young, Grant Ingram, and Lise Swartz. There was a large supporting cast, including Russell's wife, Yvonne Willier, the families of the authors, and the patients treated during the course of our investigation.

Russell Willier is in his late thirties. The stereotype of a medicine man suggests a much older person, perhaps with long grey hair, a wise and wrinkled countenance, and a spiritual detachment from the everyday world and all its trappings. This image is shattered by an introduction to this Woods Cree healer. Russell's charismatic presence makes an immediate impact. His love of people is obvious, and his energetic, outgoing nature, his warmth, and his sometimes mischievous sense of humour make it seem that one has known him for a much longer time than is the case.

Russell Willier is equally at home in front of an audience of medical anthropology students or presiding over a sweat-lodge ceremony. It is Russell's strongly held belief that, to do his job, a medicine man must be able to communicate with each person at his or her own level. To do this he must develop the ability to deal with people from all walks of life and in any situation that may present itself, a skill that Russell believes he must continually work at in order to remain a successful healer. The authors were amazed at the number and range of people whom Russell Willier knows. The healer is aware of the effect of his presence on others, and indeed jokes that he is the 'spark' of the Sucker Creek Reserve and that when he goes away for a time things are somehow not the same. Whether people approve or disapprove of Russell, agree or disagree with him, his presence is difficult to ignore.

Russell was born on the Sucker Creek Reserve. He grew up in a large family of twelve brothers and sisters. His parents worked hard to ensure that the children would be able successfully to follow the Sweetgrass Trail. Russell's father was a skilled hunter and trapper, among other things, thoroughly acquainted with the traditional Woods Cree way of life. During his childhood and young adulthood Russell had considerable experience in both native and non-native cultures. He attended Catholic mission school, then quit in order to help out on the family farm. He has worked at a variety of jobs in the larger community and on the reserve. Russell Willier's decision – and commitment – to become a healer were not easily made. As a young boy he had an unusually strong interest in and love of the natural world. When others of his age were still asleep, Russell was out exploring and observing nature. He did not think of his behaviour as out of the ordinary, but others in his family saw it as a sign of a potential to heal. Although Russell was in line to receive a medicine bundle from his great-grandfather, Moostoos, he adopted the role of medicine man by a circuitous route. Russell lived the 'wild life' for a period before his interest turned in the direction of healing. He was about thirty years old when he decided to become a medicine man.

In many ways Russell Willier is a self-taught healer. He did not serve an apprenticeship under one teacher in the traditional way. Much of his knowledge about the contents of the medicine bundle was obtained from several medicine men in the area. In the course of learning his calling, Russell has been willing to incorporate knowledge from many different sources. His willingness to learn and his ability to innovate have remained with him. He is continually seeking new and better methods to add to his healing repertoire. In his view, the role of medicine man entails a learning process that will continue throughout the course of his life.

Russell Willier's willingness to talk about his work has evolved gradually. A non-native cannot simply approach a healer and expect him or her to talk freely. Russell's co-operation was gained only after a long period of trust-building. This process was initiated by David Young while documenting traditional hide-tanning methods. (Russell, it should be noted, is trained in the Woods Cree way of tanning hides and is a skilled hunter, trapper, and professional guide.) As trust and friendship developed, Russell gradually began to talk about his involvement with native culture and religion. In 1984 the healer agreed to participate in an experiment involving treatment of non-native psoriasis sufferers in an Edmonton clinic. Russell's decision to share aspects of his knowledge with non-natives is not without risks. He faces criticism and possible ridicule from the non-native medical establishment and at the same time is open to condemnation from some members of the native community for disclosing what they consider to be secret, sacred knowledge. More seriously, he also runs the risk that he or someone close to him will be the object of a 'curse' emanating from bad medicine men.

Though aware of the risks, Russell believes that what he is trying to accomplish is important enough to warrant 'challenging the system.' He is concerned that Indian medicine is in danger of being lost as elders pass away and young people lose interest in their heritage. Russell hopes to demonstrate the efficacy of native medicine to a wider audience. He believes this will help revive a sense of pride in native young people and will stimulate their interest in native medicine and culture. He would like to 'open up some doors' for other native healers across Canada so they can practise medicine without fear of harassment. As the power of native medicine to heal becomes better known, he hopes that charlatans and bad medicine men will be exposed and 'weeded out.'

David Young is a professor in the Department of Anthropology, University of Alberta. He began teaching there in 1970, after receiving his doctorate from Stanford University. His present research and teaching interests lie in psychology, cognition, aesthetics, material culture, Japan, and the anthropology of medicine, with an emphasis on indigenous healing systems. He has done field-work in Mexico, Japan, Montana, and northern Alberta and has initiated a research project in China to examine the extent to which minority medical systems have survived there. Of all the research he has conducted to date, David Young has found the research with Russell Willier to be the most interesting. Indeed, the research has changed his life significantly.

Grant Ingram has his master's degree from the Department of Anthropology at the University of Alberta. He returned to school after taking a few years off to work and travel. He has travelled extensively throughout the Indian subcontinent and Latin America. He recently completed his MA dissertation, 'An Insider's View of the Woods Cree Cursing System: An Anthropological Analysis,' and plans to continue his studies in the anthropology of medicine and Canadian native people. He will do field-work with a national minority group in China in order to investigate how the Chinese government is coping with indigenous medical pluralism. Grant believes that the knowledge gained by this cross-cultural experience will be useful in modifying the present medical system in Canada, particularly as it concerns native communities in the north.

Lise Swartz is a doctoral student in the Department of Anthropology at the University of Alberta. Born in Denmark, she and her family came to Canada in 1956. She has travelled extensively, and from 1970 to 1977 lived in Israel where her two children were born. In 1984 she was invited by David Young to join the Psoriasis Research Project, on which her MA dissertation, 'A Cree Healer in Role Transition,' was based. She is currently planning to conduct field-work in Israel on traditional Bedouin medical practices and is also interested in studying Chinese medicine. Lise hopes to develop a research and teaching career in medical anthropology.

THE SETTING

The setting is Alberta, Canada, in the years 1984 through 1989. The specific locales are the Sucker Creek Reserve in northern Alberta, the home of Russell Willier, and Edmonton, the home of the authors and the location of the Boyle McCauley Health Centre where many of the patients described in the book were treated. To understand Russell Willier's role in the drama, it is necessary to sketch in the background of Indian medicine in Alberta and describe how Russell Willier fits into this tradition.

Before the coming of Europeans the medicine man had a position of power and status. In the words of Harold Cardinal, 'In a modern white village he would be a combination of the mayor, the local general practitioner and the local minister of the only church in town. He was the renaissance man of the Indian society.' When the first European settlers came, many of them recognized the ability of the medicine man and frequently turned to him for help. But when it became apparent to those in power that the medicine man would be the principal barrier to assimilating Indians into Anglo-Canadian society, steps were taken to weaken his influence. Missionaries, wittingly or unwittingly, aided in this task by usurping the healing role. Missionaries had considerable power in their local communities and were often able to assume the role of doctor as well as preacher. Traditional healers were subjected to criticism and abuse. Many were jailed; some were executed – and native medicine was driven underground. In time, the medicine bundles became museum pieces. To this day many Indians are secretive about native medicine and religion.

Big Joe, who died in 1987, was a native of Grouard, Alberta, a Métis settlement near the Sucker Creek Reserve and one of the oldest towns in the province. One night while sitting around a campfire on the shores of Lesser Slave Lake with Russell Willier and the authors, Big Joe described the persecution of Indian medicine and religion.

Lise: 'When they first came, the fathers with the religion about Jesus and the Bible, how did the Indians accept it?'

Big Joe: 'Not bad at the start. They accepted the religion because the Indian's God was there in the Bible and the priests tried to explain things in a nice way. So the Indians agreed, but they didn't quit their own ways. They continued to put on dances in the spring and fall where they would prophesy about things such as whether it was going to be a hard or good winter. They lived in wooden tipis at that time. Eventually more of the priests settled and built their churches. Sometimes Indians would hang a drum or a piece of ribbon in the church. The priest would walk in and say, "You can't do that," grab the object, and burn it. A lot of people didn't agree with that kind of behaviour, but they wouldn't say anything, and they let the priests do what they liked. The priests made a mistake. They never should have bothered the Indians. Indians could have made a good living today if the priests hadn't spoiled their way of life.'

Lise: 'Can you tell me about what the medicine was like then?'

Big Joe: 'People got sick and they boiled roots. I can't tell you the roots because I don't know. Although the people didn't talk or write about it, they knew their roots. They'd leave a little tobacco, dig out the root, and boil it.'

Lise: 'Could they cure everything?'

Big Joe: 'Lots of things. A lot of people got cured. It was pretty good medicine to the old people. But they are different now. They have a different religion. They don't know what the hell they're doing.'

One of the most respected of the old-time medicine men was Russell Willier's great-grandfather, Moostoos. According to the stories that have been passed down, Moostoos was one of the few medicine men with enough power to kill a 'wittigo,' an evil creature created of ice, straw, or dirt by a bad medicine man. On one occasion, a wittigo appeared in the area to attack Moostoos. Medicine men in the vicinity knew the wittigo was in their area and that individually they would not be able to defeat it. So six of them banded together and forced the wittigo to land in their midst. All six of them tackled the wittigo, which looked like a person. But after it had been captured, it coughed up several icicles that wouldn't melt. The belief was that the only person who could melt the icicles was the one the wittigo intended to attack. None of the other healers could melt the icicles, yet when Moostoos took hold of the icicles they immediately melted, at which point Moostoos killed the wittigo with an axe.

Moostoos was well known for his shaking tipi ceremony. After marking out a circle approximately six feet in diameter where the tipi was to be constructed, he gathered short pieces (about twelve inches long) of young willow or saskatoon berry bush, sharpened them to a point, and stuck them half-way into the ground inside the circle about half an inch apart until the bottom of the circle was covered with skewers. Then, around the circumference of that area, he stuck in the ground thirty or so two-inch-thick willow, poplar, or spruce saplings, leaving a narrow gap for a doorway. The poles, which extended approximately seven feet above the ground, were covered with three moose hides. The poles were bunched together at the top and tied with a couple of leather thongs. One or two rattles were tied to the leather thongs holding down the moose hide. When the tipi was ready, Moostoos would be tied with his hands behind his back. Leather thongs were wound tightly around his body, he was covered with a blanket, and more thongs were wound around the blanket. He was then placed outside the entrance to the tipi.

The ceremony would begin, accompanied by praying and chanting. As many as two to three hundred people might be present. All of a sudden Moostoos would fly through the doorway, the tipi would begin to shake violently, the rattles would fly rapidly along the leather thongs to which they were attached, and spirits would begin speaking from different spots in the air around where the people were sitting. Hearing the cry of an eagle or other animal sounds, people would turn in the direction of the sound, but they would not see anything. Then the blanket and the leather thongs would come flying out of the tipi, and Moostoos would emerge free of all bonds.

Moostoos, in addition to performing many miraculous feats, was a powerful healer who passed his medicine bundle to Russell Willier's grandfather, who in turn passed it on to Russell's father, who died in 1987. Although Russell's father learned how to use some of the herbs in the bundle, he never became a full medicine man. When he was about seventeen, Russell inherited the medicine bundle. In it he found herbs tied together in the right combinations to be used for herbal remedies. Also included were several sacred ritual objects. When Russell was in his mid-twenties and 'felt ready,' he began to study the curative powers of plants. This meant consulting the elders for information on what parts of the plants to use, where to find them, and the best time to harvest. Much of this information was obtained from his father and from medicine men and elders in the area.

As Russell relates, 'These medicine men were actually hiding from society. They'd only come out for people who would call them when really in trouble. When the doctors couldn't do anything, the medicine man would show up and do the doctoring. This happened on and off through different parts of the reserve and also on other reserves. As things got rolling, I realized that there were medicine men, that they were there for a purpose, and that they had the power. I realized, however, that it was dying out. But, hopefully, we can turn that around. That was one of the important decisions I made when I was a young man.'

Russell Willier doctored part-time, along with his other occupations, and gradually became recognized as a medicine man. He has been notably successful in curing skin diseases, migraine headaches, and backaches. In 1980 an incident occurred that Russell describes as a miracle. The incident caused him to become fully aware of the potential of native medicine and of his own power. The patient was his mother, who, according to Russell, was diagnosed by doctors as having a 'burst stomach' that could not be cured. A Catholic priest was called in to administer the last rites, and it was agreed that Russell could take his mother home to die. For three days and nights Russell treated her with prayers and herbs. She recovered. Russell then decided that if people could be saved from such close calls he 'might as well keep on doctoring instead of hiding the saddles.' Russell Willier had become a medicine man.

SACRED WORLD-VIEW

One of the conclusions that readers will no doubt come to is that an individual like Russell Willier who has a sacred world-view invests an enormous amount of effort in its interpretation. He experiences his dreams as indications of the 'way things are moving,' and he perceives meaningful signs in events that some people would consider trivial. The essence of Russell's world-view is that nothing happens by chance. All things in the world are interrelated and mutually influence each other. If one knows how to 'read the signs,' the future may be predicted. This does not necessarily imply a deterministic world. If one perceives 'how things are moving,' action can be taken and the course of events changed. People are the victims of fate only when they do not understand how to react to the 'pattern' in the things happening around them.

The ability to understand what is happening and to act in a way that changes the future course of events entails power. A man of power like Russell Willier, however, is humble about the source of his power. As Russell likes to repeat, 'a person by himself is worth less than a blade of grass.' The power of understanding the 'way things are moving' and the power to act in a way that changes things comes ultimately from the Great Spirit, mediated by numerous good and bad spirit helpers. The world is a battleground between those who wield good and bad power and a testing ground for those who are caught between. Although there is a design to be read in everything that happens, it was not set in motion by a creator who has stepped back to watch predestination unfold. The design is constantly changing, like clouds blowing in the wind, as women and men exercise their knowledge.

The authors had read accounts of the sacred world-view in studies of remote tribes in Africa and South America, but we did not suspect that this kind of world-view could be found so close to home until we met Russell Willier. We found a world-view right on our doorsteps that could hardly be more different in many respects from the one to which we were accustomed. Most non-natives, particularly those living in the city, have no idea that an alternative cosmology exists and thrives in our technological society; however, native people like Russell Willier are well aware of Western cosmology with its split between mind and matter. He knows that most non-natives would view him as being superstitious, but from his point of view most non-natives are ignorant of and insensitive to the meaning of what is happening around them. Non-natives, he believes, cannot hope to achieve wisdom if they 'can't see what is in front of their own eyes.'

Russell Willier has an open, receptive attitude towards life, an attitude that seems to be shared by many native people. They believe that each person has the right and obligation to live in accordance with his or her own world-view. Each person, moreover, has the right to ask the spirits for help. Spirits reveal meaning to individuals through their dreams and through the pattern of events that unfold. Thus, no ideology or dogma can be valid for everyone. Native religion emphasizes the priesthood of all believers. Nobody has the right to challenge the authenticity of another's spiritual experiences.

This means that there cannot be a single belief system for a group of native people even if they belong to the same tribe or reserve. A group may share certain traditions, rituals, and stories, but there is no total system of meaning.

It is for this reason that this book concentrates on one person. We make no claim that this glimpse into the life and thought of Russell Willier is typical of native life and thought in general or even of Woods Cree life and thought. It may not even be typical of Russell Willier himself a few years from now. If world-views differ in many respects from one person to the next, how can one generalize about a 'shared culture'? Yet this is what many anthropologists and other social scientists do. Although members of a group necessarily share some things, much of what is considered to be the culture of a group may be nothing more than a creation of the anthropologist.

Attempting to understand another person's life and thought is not without its risks. An in-depth encounter of this sort is bound to change the investigator. Taking another world-view seriously means that we do not regard it as consisting merely of interesting beliefs. We attempt to suspend disbelief and pretend a belief is true. The more we pretend a belief is true, the more we begin to see past its form to its essence, which, in the case of a belief held by someone like Russell Willier, is often quite sophisticated. The more we feel our way into the essential nature of a variety of beliefs and see their logical connections, the more we realize that the world could in fact be like that. The belief system's internal logic appears quite convincing once it is understood and gives meaning to many things that might appear baffling in another system.

We cannot say that we have given up our Western heritage and 'gone native,' but all three of us have been changed by our encounter with Russell Willier. We frequently see or suspect a pattern where none existed before. How far can we move in this direction and still be scientists? The answer must vary with each individual. We would argue that good science involves setting up creative opposition between two or more systems so that experiences and concepts can be explored from a variety of angles. This is intended not as a reiteration of the idea that all things are relative, but as a claim that anything of importance has multiple dimensions and that a single world-view is limited in its ability to perceive and deal with more than a few of these dimensions. One does not have to give up one world-view in order to enter into another. We have learned that it is valuable to let world-views interact and to allow ourselves to be stimulated and enriched by the experiences that result from that interaction.

In the next chapter we move directly to Russell Willier's conception of the cosmos and the relation between the world of humans and the spiritual world. This is the big picture that provides the context for Russell's practice as a medicine man.

❧ The Spiritual World

Russell Willier, his brother Raymond, David Young, and Grant Ingram were sitting around the table at Russell's house drinking coffee and talking about Russell's plans for building a health centre on the reserve. Ray looked out the window to see ominous black clouds rolling in. 'Holy sufferance! I should have baled my hay yesterday,' he said.

'I thought you were supposed to be able to prevent that kind of thing,' David said jokingly to Russell. 'I remember you had lots of trouble with haying last year, didn't you?'

'Right through till Christmas. I and another guy went to the fields and loaded the hay on a flat deck with a fork. Coming home we had two flat tires on the same side.' He laughed.

'I guess Indians are not supposed to make hay.'

'Indians are not supposed to make money, period.' He laughed again.

'Guess I'd better get home,' Ray said. After he had left, we continued talking for a few minutes. It got darker, and Russell said he should get out and try to do something, as protecting the hayfields was part of his job. We went outside and Russell began looking for an axe. We thought he was going to sacrifice one of the geese running around the yard. He couldn't find the axe.

'I've got a knife. We can use it instead of the axe,' Russell said. He lit a fungus as incense and placed it in a lid on top of an upended log. He stuck the edge of the knife blade in the rim of the log, as if he were preparing to split it. The tip of the knife extended beyond the top of the log to point directly at the centre of the approaching storm. Russell began to pray loudly in Cree. He faced the storm. His words were almost drowned out by the crash of thunder and lightning. It was an impressive scene.

After the ceremony, Russell explained that the knife should split the storm, with some of the clouds moving off to one side of the blade and the rest moving off to the other side. He said, however, that he was a little late. The storm should have been caught when it was still distant. He explained that if he had been outside instead of inside having coffee he would have seen the storm in time. Yet he hoped the ceremony would have some effect.

We jumped into Russell's pick-up truck and headed for the hayfields to see if the ceremony would work. Russell raced down the drive, took a left turn onto a rutted road that went past the band offices, and eventually turned off the road to follow car tracks through a grassy area interspersed with shallow sloughs and patches of poplar. Although the hayfields were only about four miles from Russell's house as the crow flies, the track followed a circuitous route, and it took us more than half an hour to reach the edge of the hayfields. As we bounced along, occasionally hitting our heads on the ceiling of the cab, we continued to talk.

Finally, Russell stopped the truck and turned it around to face the storm. 'The storm's coming this way,' he said. 'Pretty dark up there, but it's beginning to split. We'll get half an hour of rain, but that's not bad compared to what they're getting over there.' It appeared to be much darker on either side of us. The light drumming of the rain on the roof of the cab made a pleasant sound. In about fifteen minutes the rain stopped. It looked as though we were in a huge black tunnel, with solid black clouds dropping down to touch the earth many miles away on either side of us.

'Axes do a better job. That's what my dad usually used, a double-bladed axe. But I broke mine.' He was smiling.

'Does the North Wind help split the clouds?' one of us asked.

'Yeah, the winds help.'

'How are the Grandfathers connected with the winds?'

'Well, the Great Spirit has helpers like Fire, Thunder, Wind, and Water. They are the elements – the Grandfathers.'

'How many Grandfathers are there?'

'There are lots of Grandfathers, but these are the main ones. We don't have anything written down in black and white like the Bible. But we use the Bible for reference. For example, when Jesus was being crucified, the Grandfathers, such as Thunder and Earthquake, were there to help him. All he had to do was ask, but he didn't ask. They made a lot of noise, but he still didn't ask.'

'Were the Grandfathers here when the world was created?'

'Right from the beginning. And it has always been the same. They're there to help, but you've got to ask. If you don't ask them, how are they going to help you?'

'Are there lots of other Grandfathers besides the elemental spirits?'

'Right. There are the animal spirits but they're not half as strong as the elemental spirits like Thunder. You can't picture how powerful the elemental spirits actually are. Take Tornado, for example, or Lightning. More power is there than we can imagine, but we don't need all that power. All we need is just a little speck, and that's all we ask for.'

'You mentioned Wind as one of the Grandfather spirits. Is that split into North Wind, South Wind ... ?'

'Yes. It's actually one wind that can come in from four directions. It's all the same power.'

'Going back to the animal spirits, do the animal spirits usually appear as animals?'

'Yes. But the more powerful spirits can appear in different forms. A powerful plant spirit, for example, can talk to you.'

'Do they appear as humans?'

'Sometimes they will appear as only the top half of a human so they can talk to you. You won't see the rest.'

'Are the plant spirits Grandfathers too?'

'Yes. If you use a plant and ask that plant spirit to get help from the Great Spirit, the power will come through. That's where you get the real power.'

'How about the spirits of people who have died? They're not Grandfather spirits?'

'Most of those spirits can be used for bad purposes very easily.'

'You can't use Grandfather spirits for bad purposes?'

'It's pretty hard. If you try to use a Grandfather spirit for bad purposes, it will eventually go away and you won't be able to heal. You can't hold Grandfather spirits.'

'You can hold the spirits of the dead?'

'Yeah. You can also use them for good. If you start off using them for good and stick with it, you can't ask for better helpers.'

'If someone goes bad and the Grandfather spirits pull out, where does the person get his power after that?'

'Down below. The bad spirits will step in.'

'The bad spirits from dead people?'

'Not necessarily. Let's say a person starts using Grandfather spirits for good but he gets too greedy. He starts asking for different things, but the good spirits may back off. At that point, he would have to turn to the bad side and use the bad spirits. You'll still have the Wind helping you, for example, but it will not be the same Wind as before. It'll be another Wind from the dark side.'

'So all the Grandfather spirits have two sides, the good Wind and the bad Wind, the good Fire and the bad Fire?'

'Right, there's a split.'

'Is that the same with people who have died? Do they have the good and the bad?'

'Right.'

'If you start doing bad, do you go to the bad Grandfather spirits or the bad spirits of people who have died?'

'Either one. It's up to you. If you stay on the good side, which is more powerful, the bad spirits won't be able to touch you. But if you switch to the bad side, you automatically lose your power to heal. You're finished.'

'But the bad Grandfather spirits are more powerful than the bad spirits of people who have died?'

'Yes, the spirits of the dead are limited, but the Grandfathers' are not limited.'

'But you can't hold a bad Grandfather spirit? You can't control it?'

'You don't really have to try to hold a bad Grandfather spirit. He'll help you anyway in order to get your soul. When you die, you'll have to go the bad side.'

'What is the bad side?'

'A bad guy will probably go to a fogged area for five hundred, seven hundred, or maybe a thousand years to pay for his debt.'

'Will he get another chance?'

'He'll make it to heaven eventually. He won't go to hell. But if you're in a misty place because of what you did on earth, you can't find your way out for a long time.'

At this point Russell paused. He took a long look at the storm.

'It split. Look how dark it is over there, and over there. But the results would have been even better if I had concentrated on it. That is what I'm saying about doctoring too. If you concentrate on the people as they're coming in to be healed, the results seem to be a lot better. If you have to do too many different kinds of things to make a living, you can't concentrate on healing and the results are not as good.'

'Going back to the spirits, do many people around here think the way you do?'

'Not that many. They may have an idea about the spirits, but unless they're raised with it they don't know that much. Lots of people don't want to get involved because the only time they hear about Indian medicine is when somebody got jinxed and a person died. They don't hear the good side of Indian medicine, especially the younger people.'

'If a plant spirit appears to you, is there any way to know whether it's one of the minor plant spirits or one of the powerful Grandfather spirits who has appeared as a plant? Can you tell the difference?'

'It'll tell you.'

'So the powerful spirits can appear in different forms?'

'The spirits can appear in any form you want. But they don't necessarily talk to you right away. They may watch for a long time until they feel you are capable of understanding. That's when they'll talk to you. The Grandfather spirits are not like the spirits of the dead, which are on the dangerous side. Really, people shouldn't monkey around with the dead. It's not their type of work. If someone is in the foggy area, how are you going to get him to work for you on the good side? He's thinking about getting out of his situation, right?'

'What if you knew someone was a great healer who had died, like your grandfather, Moostoos? Could you go to his spirit for help?'

'I don't know. We do ask for his assistance to a certain extent, but we don't try to hold him. To hold a spirit, he has to be with you constantly. That's a little different than what I'm doing.'

'Can you ask the Grandfather spirits for assistance at any time, or are some spirits too powerful at certain times of the year?'

'It doesn't really matter when you ask for it. Power is power. I remember one episode when there were no clouds, and yet we asked the Thunder Spirit to come. In doing this, we had to have lots of faith. The Thunder heard our prayers and came. It was a lot louder than what we heard today. It shook the ground, but there were no clouds, only a blue sky. There were some witnesses, some white people from Calgary who never believed that anything like that could happen. They said they would have a lot of respect for Indian religion from that time on. It opened their minds right then and there. They saw the power come through.'

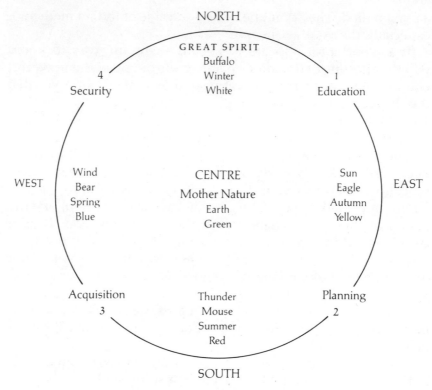

NORTH

GREAT SPIRIT
Buffalo
Winter
White

4
Security

1
Education

WEST

Wind
Bear
Spring
Blue

CENTRE
Mother Nature
Earth
Green

Sun
Eagle
Autumn
Yellow

EAST

Acquisition
3

Thunder
Mouse
Summer
Red

Planning
2

SOUTH

Russell Willier's Version of Native Cosmology

After talking a while longer we drove on to where a friend of Russell's was baling hay. He was sitting in his truck having a cup of coffee, as it was raining a little, but it had not rained hard enough to stop work for the day. After talking to Russell the man resumed his baling, and we drove back to Russell's house.

COSMOLOGY

The preceding conversation was edited to omit extraneous material and to make it easier to read. In a few cases the material was slightly rearranged or a few words added, for the sake of clarity. This involves some interpretation, obviously, but its purpose is to convey the meaning of what was said as faithfully as possible. The advantage of a narrative of this sort is that it provides a context for the various cosmological ideas that were raised during the conversation.

We will now expand upon these ideas by pulling together material from a variety of contexts. We will also bring in things that Russell said or did on other occasions. The material has been selected and arranged by the authors, and there is more room for interpretation. First, let's examine Russell's beliefs concerning the spirits.

Because of their wrongdoing, people are less worthy than a blade of grass to talk to the Great Spirit directly. There is a spiritual level between humans and the Great Spirit composed of the elemental Grandfather spirits, animal spirits (including animals, birds, and insects), plant spirits, and the spirits of rocks. Any of these spirits can be either good or bad. The good spirits are the helpers and messengers of the Great Spirit and also can be invited by humans to assist with a variety of tasks. Direct approaches to the Great Spirit are made only in matters pertaining to the salvation of one's soul and tend to occur more frequently as people near death. The Great Spirit is the only one with the authority to determine a person's fate.

There are primary elemental spirits such as Thunder, Wind, Earth, and Sun, as well as a spirit for every species of animal, bird, and insect on the earth. Every living creature is a tangible expression of the spirit for that species. Living creatures are put on the earth to supply food and medicine for human beings. For this reason, a spirit such as the bear spirit is not upset when individual bears are killed for a good purpose. The only expectation is that an offering will be left if the slain animal is to be used for medicine. In fact, if a particular species is not utilized, it may be taken away. When individual animals are killed their souls go to another world, which in Russell's opinion is like a big-game park. There they wait until there is a need for them in the world of humans, at which point they take on material form.

These individual souls should not be confused with the primordial animal spirits that assist the Great Spirit.

Some animal spirits are more important for specific medicine men than others. For Russell, the primary animal spirits are the eagle, the bear, and the buffalo. Other important spirits are the wild goose, the skunk, the porcupine, the beaver, the weasel, the elk, and the horse. Like the elemental spirits, animal spirits cannot be controlled. They can be invited to a sweat-lodge ceremony, for example, but they cannot be forced to enter. What spirit is invited depends on the need of the medicine man. The eagle is called upon when the medicine man is in need of wisdom, particularly the wisdom to interpret the past or to see the future. A specific spirit may also be invited to assist in curing when an animal part of that species has been used in preparing the medicine. Thus, if a bear gall-bladder has been used in a medicinal combination the bear spirit may be invited to assist in the healing.

Spirits can appear in a variety of forms. The elemental Grandfather spirits generally appear in natural form and are free to appear at any time. For example, if Thunder is called, it may come regardless of weather conditions, sometimes putting in a violent appearance on a day with sunshine and white clouds. Animal and plant spirits may appear as animals or plants, or they may appear as humans. In a sweat-lodge ceremony an eagle may make its presence known by flapping around inside the sweat-lodge, or a bear may sniff in someone's face. Plant spirits often take on human form to facilitate communication. The better one is prepared to meet the spirits the more clearly their presence will be perceived. Fasting and prayer may be required for deep communication with the spirit world, but even simple purification rites such as burning sweetgrass or a fungus from the diamond willow will allow one to perceive the presence of spirits. Russell claims that burning incense is like opening a curtain. When the curtain has been pulled back one can see and communicate directly with the spirits. The spirit can be seen with such clarity that it may be difficult to tell whether the visitor is a spirit or a real animal. The spirit may communicate in a human voice; when this happens, the experience may deeply frighten all but the most courageous. Alternatively, a spirit may appear to a person who is sleeping or who has entered a trance. The visitation is then referred to as a vision and has some of the qualities of a dream. Dreaming is considered very important, and dreams may be carefully told to family members and discussed around the breakfast table.

Spirits may be called upon for a variety of reasons. They may be asked to assist in healing ceremonies; they may provide spiritual guidance to the healer and to believers assembled in a sweat-lodge; they may help a medicine man see the future in a rattle ceremony; they may even be asked to change the course of future events in some way. The role of the spirits in healing and sweat-lodge ceremonies will be discussed later in this book. The role of spirits in helping individuals look into or change the future is illustrated in the examples that follow.

In 1987 David Young and his family were invited to a rattle ceremony conducted by a close associate of Russell Willier's, a shaman from a nearby reserve. The ceremony, which appears to be a variant of the shaking tipi, was conducted in the shaman's large log house, with more than sixty people in attendance. An elaborate altar lay on buffalo skins in the middle of the immense, open-beamed living-room. The altar consisted of flags of different colours stuck in a tub of sand, cloth prints of various colours, several pipes, tobacco, food offerings, rattles, and eagle wings. The entire altar area was enclosed by a string to which had been tied tiny pouches of tobacco several inches apart. Before the ceremony, individuals went to the kitchen to present the shaman with prints, tobacco, and gifts, and to ask about something for which they were seeking a specific answer.

The men and boys sat on one side of the altar, the women and girls on the other. After everyone was seated in the living-room the shaman entered. A group of four elders sat at one end of the altar area and three singers sat at the other. Helpers nailed blankets over the door, and those present were asked to remove their wallets and any metal objects.

The shaman lighted pieces of fungus. He proceeded to purify

himself and the altar area. He then delivered a sermon in both Cree and English, warning participants that to enter into the ceremony with less than complete sincerity would endanger the shaman's life. He warned that those with an insincere heart would be removed from the building by the spirits and would find themselves outside in the dark. All who wished to were invited to leave. The shaman filled the stone pipes with tobacco and smoked them one by one, after which individuals were selected to stand at each corner of the altar area. The shaman was tied securely hand and foot with leather thongs, wrapped in a blanket, tied again with thongs, and laid face-down in the middle of the altar area. The shaman was moaning loudly, as his hands had been tied behind his back with his thumbs severely bent. The lights were turned out and the congregation found themselves in total darkness.

The shaman announced that he would go into a trance and enter the spirit world, but that he would return at the end of the ceremony provided there were no sceptics in the room. He said the spirits would soon be arriving to check everything out. If everything had been done properly they would answer the questions raised by individuals prior to the ceremony and would also accept questions from the floor. The singers began to drum and chant loudly. Before long, the spirits began to enter the room. Rattles flashed like fireflies and flew around the room. Animal and bird spirits made a variety of snorting and crying sounds. One by one the spirits possessed the shaman. They spoke to the congregation, encouraging them to ask questions. The shaman spoke in different voices, depending on the spirit who had possessed him, and a helper translated the messages from Cree to English. Although the ceremony was awesome, to say the least, it was occasionally punctuated by humour. The Joking Spirit announced in a loud voice that the ladies had better watch out, as the handsomest man in the world had arrived. Some laughed and joked with the spirit.

From time to time a spirit would repeat a question that some-one had asked before the ceremony and would then proceed to answer it. Russell Willier, who was standing in one corner, had asked a question about his mother, who was critically ill in the hospital as a result of a curse and a subsequent car accident. He was told that she would be assisted by spirit healers. In fact, they were at that very moment on the way to the hospital, where they would remain for four days. Everyone voiced approval, and Russell thanked the spirit. The spirit announced that it was breaking a long string of curses that had been inflicted upon Russell and his relatives. Russell expressed great relief, saying that he would be able to sleep well for the first time in many months.

When a spirit known as the Healing Doctor entered, some members of the congregation made requests concerning the health of loved ones. If the sick person was in attendance at the ceremony, the spirit would perform healing on the spot, indicating his presence by an action such as pressing down hard on the top of the person's head. If the sick person was not in attendance the Healing Doctor would announce the outcome of the illness. Other spirits answered questions on the success of business enterprises and other matters of deep concern. Although people were packed into the room, sitting so close to each other on the floor that it was barely possible to move, the spirits moved silently among the congregation, indicating their presence in a variety of ways. For example, I was bumped hard on the head several times with a rattle, and my wife and daughters heard a mouse squeaking at their feet.

The ceremony eventually came to an end, and the lights came on. The shaman was found, untied but still wrapped in the blanket, at the back of the room on the side occupied by the men and boys. He appeared to be in a daze and said very little. The food offerings were passed around and consumed, and one by one members of the congregation thanked the shaman and left quietly.

Spirits can assist the shaman not only in foretelling but in changing the future. One of Russell's teachers, a medicine man more than ninety years old who lives alone in the bush, practises court magic. Using his inner eye and assisted by certain plants, this hermit specializes in visualizing the courtroom scene of an impending trial. Having seen what will transpire and what will be said, he is in a position to advise a client about what steps to take to avoid an unfavourable judgment. This assistance is provided only when the shaman believes that a judgment would be unjust or otherwise detrimental to the rehabilitation of an individual.

Another way in which spirits can be asked to change the course of future events is to use them for bad medicine. This will be discussed in a later chapter. The status of bad spirits in Russell's belief system is unclear. On the one hand, ultimate power resides with the Great Spirit, in that a coalition of Grandfathers and the Great Spirit is able to defeat the power of any combination of evil spirits in the cosmos. On the other hand, evil continues to exist and seems to be constantly fuelled by the evil in the human mind. It would be too strong to say that human nature is essentially evil, but it is no exaggeration to say that people are often tempted to seek personal gain by illicit means. Although justice is ultimately assured, the road to goodness is narrow and difficult to follow. The road to ill-gotten fame and fortune may be a dead end, but it is broad and easy to follow.

With the exception of the Great Spirit, each good spirit has an evil counterpart. The good elemental spirits are somewhat unpredictable and uncontrollable and difficult to work with. Their evil counterparts, however, are readily available and eager to serve. Sometimes temptation is too great, especially in a moment of anger or greed, and even a good medicine man may give in and seek the assistance of an evil spirit. The effect is usually immediately gratifying, with the consequence that the medicine man finds it increasingly easy to rely on evil power. In this way he is soon hooked and may spend the rest of his days practising black magic. Once a medicine man has dabbled in the black arts, his soul can still be saved by the Great Spirit, but he is no longer any good for healing.

Calling upon good spirits can lead to disaster under certain conditions. It is risky, for example, to call upon the North Wind in the winter when it is at the height of its power. Like the other spirits, the North Wind has specific qualities that can be the source of both strength and weakness. The North Wind tends to be impatient, and if called upon in the winter when its power is overflowing it may go beyond what has been requested. If the North Wind has been called upon to send back a curse, it may do so with such vehemence that the curse may kill its original sender. Indeed, there may be a fine line between sending and returning a curse. The danger of using an impatient power is increased if the medicine man himself is impatient. Russell Willier, who perceives himself to be impatient, prefers to 'lie low' in the winter when any call for assistance may be answered by the North Wind.

There are also occasions when a medicine man may be particularly vulnerable to possession by evil spirits, for example, during the process of obtaining the shaking tipi, which Russell hopes to do in the near future. This process involves a vision quest in pursuit of power that will reside permanently in one's body so that there is no need to rely exclusively upon the assistance of uncontrollable, and therefore unpredictable, spirits. The shaman must fast in a circle of power for four days and nights, preferably in a high place. At the end of each day the vision quester goes down to a sweat-lodge that is being tended by another shaman who already has the shaking tipi. The vision quester relates his experiences of the day to the other shaman who, with the aid of the spirits, provides interpretation. The most hazardous time is the fourth and final day. The sweat must be completed before sundown; otherwise, instead of the desired protector spirit, evil spirits might come and inhabit the vision quester's body. From that day forward the quester would have to serve as a bad medicine man. He would not necessarily be identifiable as bad, because it would not be prudent for him to relate what happened. The quester is also vulnerable through his shaman associate. An evil shaman can allow the quester to do all the work and then steal the power that has been gained.

An interesting characteristic of spirits is that they try to entice the vision quester to enter the spirit world with them. When the spirits appear during a vision quest, the quester should have with him something concrete like a coyote tail as a reminder of the natural world, because the temptation the spirits have to offer is possibly the greatest ever encountered. The spirits may come in other forms – an old man, an old lady, or a bear, for example. If an old lady comes, it is easy to forget that she is a spirit. If she asks you to go with her and you do, your spirit leaves your body and may not be able to get back. The vision quester would then be found dead that night. A whole family of spirits might come and adopt the quester as a grandson. This would make it especially tempting to go through the 'doorway' with the spirits and to forget all responsibilities.

To illustrate the dangers of entering deeply into the spiritual world, Russell told of one man who was seeking a vision in order to see his real self. The man was visited by the Eagle Spirit. The Eagle Spirit asked the man to come with him, and the man was taken to a ledge high up in the Rocky Mountains. The ledge was only a few feet wide, overlooking a drop of several thousand feet. This was especially frightening for the man because his greatest fear was of heights. Somehow the man withstood the ordeal until the Eagle returned for him.

On another occasion a man who was seeking a vision was visited by the Fire Spirit. He was frightened so badly that when he came down he had a streak of pure white in his hair. A final example is provided by a man who sought a vision on top of a mountain in Montana. He was seated in his circle of power when an old woman approached and tried to talk to him. He ignored her. He thought she was a human being until she walked into a rock and disappeared. At that point the man jumped up from his vision quest site and ran down the mountain as fast as he could. Although stories like this are told with a good deal of humour, they enhance rather than diminish the real fear that accompanies a vision quest.

Russell recently experienced being taken on a spirit journey while doing a vision quest. In the spring of 1988 he was asked by one of his clients on another reserve to prevent further harm from a powerful medicine man who had killed his daughter with a curse. This was the same medicine man who had killed Russell's father several months earlier. Russell felt he could not let the bad medicine man go unchallenged. Yet he could not send a curse of his own, as this would forever put him on the evil side. Also, to send back a curse can involve the medicine man in open warfare, in which the good medicine man must always assume a defensive role. Faced with this dilemma, Russell decided that he would have to seek wisdom from the spiritual world by participating in a vision quest. Using a site in the Swan Hills, a rugged area about an hour's drive from the reserve, Russell embarked on a four-day quest. He didn't eat or drink, and he dared not sleep as long as the sun was up. On the last day a spirit came and took him on a trip to a neighbouring province where he had a number of interesting experiences, including the experience of entering buildings by walking through walls. Russell thought he was in his natural body, but after what seemed like several days of spiritual instruction he found himself flying back to the Swan Hills and was startled to see himself sitting on the top of a hill inside his circle of tobacco where he had begun the quest. He knew then that he had experienced spirit travel and felt fortunate that he had been able to return to his body. As a result of instruction while in the spiritual world, Russell and his client were able to plan a course of action to deal with the enemy shaman.

Wittigo are some of the most fearsome evil spirits. Made of wood, ice, or mud and herbs, they assume human form and eat human flesh. It is thought that some individuals in mental institutions were possessed and turned into wittigo. If they had been allowed to remain loose they would have become cannibals because they would have had nothing else to eat. No one has been killed by wittigo in recent times but there were instances of wittago cannibalism in the late nineteenth century. Russell says that his great-grandfather, Moostoos, was renowned as a slayer of wittigo.

Harm is usually brought by evil spirits, though it can also result from the failure to perform ceremonies properly. In 1986 the Sucker Creek Band decided to hold a ceremony of thanksgiving in early October. Russell Willier shot two moose for the feast and gave them to the band to be distributed. Distribution was handled by a cousin of Russell's who took all the credit for providing the meat. The afternoon was spent in playing hand games, which were supposed to end in time for sacred offerings to be made before sundown. But people were so engrossed in playing that they forgot about the ceremonies until after the sun had set. This proved to be a costly mistake.

The ceremonies were conducted by the cousin who had distributed the meat, by an elder from the Sucker Creek Reserve, and by a visiting shaman from Saskatchewan.

That same night Russell returned home to find an owl waiting for him. Russell recognized the owl as a spirit and talked to it. The owl said that it wanted Russell's life in place of the offering that was supposed to have been given before sundown at the ceremony. Russell explained that he had nothing to do with the mistake. He said that he had killed the moose, but that the ceremony had been conducted by three others. Russell begged for mercy, saying he was too young to die. The owl screeched loudly and flew off into the darkness. Later that night the shaman from Saskatchewan received a long-distance phone call saying that his daughter had just died. The next night Russell's cousin and three friends were drinking together when one of the friends died under mysterious circumstances. A few days later the elder who had helped with the ceremony learned that his niece had died.

Russell says that many people have gotten careless about the rituals or have forgotten how to do them properly. It is, therefore, becoming more and more dangerous to participate in ceremonies – which means that many times they simply are not done. When asked about what happens if the ceremonies are not performed, Russell replied that without ceremonies people are totally unprotected and vulnerable to evil spirits. Thus, a kind of double bind exists: it is dangerous to take part in ceremonies conducted by incompetent people, but it is even more dangerous not to do the ceremonies at all. Such is the dilemma that Russell Willier constantly faces.

In Russell's mind, cosmological, ordering principles are expressed symbolically in material items such as the coloured prints that are hung in the sweat-lodge. A white cloth represents the Great Spirit, the principle of creativity, but also stands for the buffalo and for north. The buffalo in turn represents human qualities, like wisdom, and north represents winter. Yellow represents the eagle, east, autumn, and the sun. The eagle represents far-sightedness. Red represents thunder, south, summer, and mouse. Thunder represents great power, of the kind one might turn to when healing a very sick person, and mouse represents the trait of collecting material possessions.

There are two colour systems, but white, yellow, and red are the same in both systems. Blue stands for the wind in one system and for prayer in the other. Blue also stands for west, spring, and mother bear. Green stands for earth and Mother Nature, and is at the centre of life. People wishing to be doctored are requested to bring the medicine man tobacco and a print (a square metre of coloured cloth). They almost instinctively buy a print whose colour represents qualities or powers they need, depending upon the type and severity of the illness. If a person came with a dark-blue print, for example, the medicine man would ask the female black bear to doctor him. The black bear, which takes good care of its cubs, could impart some of the qualities of being a good parent to the patient.

These cosmological principles are important for understanding two major concepts employed by Russell: the 'Sweetgrass Trail' and the 'Medicine Wheel' or 'Medicine Circle.' The Sweetgrass Trail is explained in terms of the different 'roads' that people take on their journey through life. The central road is likened to a tree trunk, and an individual can diverge from it at any time. A person can also veer away for a period, as in drinking or drug use, and later return to the Sweetgrass Trail. There is no guarantee, however, that a person will reach the culmination of his or her journey. A person can make it nearly all the way by attaining the age of seventy or over and still experience a sudden heart attack. Accidents or mishaps can cause others to fall off the path at a very early age. The various branches leading off the main road are many, some leading to death in the form of cancer, brain tumours, or AIDS, and others to liver problems or suicide.

If the proper road is adhered to and an individual reaches the age of eighty to one hundred, the Sweetgrass Trail has been successfully followed and fulfilment has been achieved. At this point death is not to be feared. On the Sweetgrass Trail the good years start at about the age of fifty.

Bound together with that of the Sweetgrass Trail is the concept of the Medicine Circle. According to Russell, all people emit certain colours of light at different times in their lives. This is their Medicine Circle. The shade of colour that a person radiates depends on where they are in terms of closing the circle. When the circle is broken, a distinct colour of light is emitted. Russell believes that the lights people give off can only be revealed when tobacco is offered during a healing ceremony.

The four cardinal directions are of great importance in understanding the Medicine Circle. The four directions divide the Medicine Circle into four quadrants, each symbolizing a component necessary for a person's life. The first quadrant represents education, occupation, or special skill; the second, far-sightedness and the ability to plan ahead. The third quadrant stands for material possessions, home, and spouse, and the last symbolizes the happiness that comes from family life and having children.

The association between these qualities essential to self-fulfilment and specific animals is obvious to Russell. The eagle, for example, flies high and sees great distances, the mouse is well known as a collector, and the bear is recognized for its maternal qualities. Each segment of the Medicine Circle is important in its own right, but the parts must work in harmony for a person to close the circle and reach fulfilment. At a very early age, a child cannot have the Eagle Spirit's ability to plan ahead, but it does have the Buffalo Spirit's ability to learn. The child of course will start to roam a little and will begin to develop the Eagle Spirit. Eventually the Mouse Spirit will become active, and the child will acquire a few possessions. The child may also begin to develop a good heart, a quality that will become important later when she or he grows up and raises a family. The child thus begins to develop qualities associated with all four segments of the Medicine Circle, even though these qualities will not attain their full potential until later in life. The most important thing is for parents to help the child explore all four segments early in life.

There can be any combination of the four quadrants of the Medicine Circle in a person's life. The segments are ultimately connected, and a deficiency in one area has an influence on the rest of the circle. To understand how the Medicine Circle works as a whole it is necessary to consider the examples that Russell used to explain two different lives.

One example is provided by the man who loves to chase women. He will spend all his money on women, failing to acquire possessions (Mouse Spirit). He won't plan ahead (Eagle Spirit), and won't have a family (Bear Spirit). So the circle is not closed. This will eventually have negative consequences for his job. At the age of fifty when life should bring great fulfilment this man will be unhappy.

Russell cited his father as an example of a Medicine Circle that is unbroken. Before his death in 1987 he was in his eighties and had fathered twelve children. Over his lifetime he attained a balance of the four essential elements, namely, buffalo, eagle, mouse, and bear. He could go to any one of his children for assistance because they were all raised properly on the Sweetgrass Trail. He had nothing to fear in this life or the afterworld. He had closed his circle and reached fulfilment.

It is clear that the Medicine Circle and the Sweetgrass Trail are virtually the same thing. To reach fulfilment in life one has to follow the Sweetgrass Trail and to follow the Sweetgrass Trail successfully one has to close the Medicine Circle. Variations on this basic theme encompass the entire range of human conditions.

To return to the main theme of this chapter, Russell Willier conceives of the cosmos as one in which little happens by chance. Although evil may seem to prosper in the short term, in the long term individuals suffer the consequences of their actions. Illnesses and mishaps that appear accidental to the Western mind are in many cases the results of a person's failure to develop a healthy life-style or a balanced approach to living. In other cases misfortune is due to malevolent intent on the part of others, but even this is usually due to impropriety of some sort, such as attracting envy through the display of wealth. What the Buddhist would call 'karmic tendencies' inherited from past actions are the primary contributing factors to one's character and are thus expressed in everything a person does. Internal character is also expressed in one's energy field, which is invisible to most but can be 'read' by a medicine man. To the extent that one is able to change one's actions, it is possible to alter one's character and, ultimately, one's constitution and ability to resist illness and misfortune. Although native religion with its emphasis on spirits may appear irrational or superstitious to many non-natives, it rests on a basic affirmation that the world is orderly and governed by cause-and-effect relations. Less is attributed to chance than in many non-native belief systems.

The cosmos is also a personal one. The forces of nature and the principles they represent are capable of being visualized in human form. Nature cannot be controlled, yet it is possible to live one's life sufficiently in accordance with nature that communication with abstract forces and principles is possible. Being tuned in to nature is the ultimate source of power and self-fulfilment. On the other side of the coin, the forces of evil in the universe are constantly fed by human characteristics such as greed and jealousy.

Some literature on traditional non-Western religions emphasizes the use of magic to control the forces of nature. This emphasis does not do justice to any complex belief system. Magic may be used on occasion by a medicine man to impress an audience, but it plays little role in dealing with the forces of nature, which must be approached with appropriate awe and supplication. Non-natives tend to view native descriptions of encounters with animal spirits as childish, to say the least. This view fails to take into account the rich symbolism of native religion. It would be inaccurate to think that someone like Russell Willier does not distinguish between the content of a vision and the reality that lies behind it. The principle of wisdom in the universe may take the form of a living buffalo or even a human being because as humans we would be unable to perceive abstract forces unclothed in flesh. Russell would agree that we create our deities in a form that we can understand. This is a feature of many religions. Because native people live in close contact with nature, it is fitting that their understanding of cosmic principles should be expressed in terms of natural creatures and phenomena.

We are emphasizing that understanding of the world-view of an individual from a different culture is possible only when some translation or interpretation is done. Beliefs that appear irrational or superstitious when taken literally are then seen to be reasonable, and sometimes extremely sophisticated, in the context of their own system. Individual beliefs or practices should not be taken out of context but should be meaningfully related to other beliefs and practices in the system. It is the system as a whole that should be judged. A belief system such as Russell Willier's can take on great significance and power, as the growing interest in native religion attests. This interest should not be regarded as a return to superstition and uncritical thinking, but as the expression of a longing for a cosmos that is orderly and responsive to the individual seeking to harmonize life and nature. Native religion is remarkably successful in providing people with a way to get in touch with their natural origins. For this reason native religion has the potential to speak to a large audience.

❦ Good and Bad Medicine

In the summer of 1986 Grant Ingram had the opportunity to live with the Russell Willier family. What follows is Grant's account of what he learned about Russell Willier's beliefs concerning the relationship between good and bad medicine.

I arrived at the Willier household on the evening of 10 June 1986 loaded down with what turned out to be mostly expendable items, such as camera equipment. My field-work was intended to complement the Psoriasis Research Project, which involved the treatment of non-native patients with psoriasis at a health clinic in Edmonton. My plan was to document Russell's treatment of psoriasis patients from his own culture and in his own setting. It turned out that no native psoriasis patients came for treatment during the course of my visit. Even if they had, it is doubtful whether I would have been allowed to observe treatment, as native patients are reluctant to allow any kind of documentation of the treatment process. Instead, I concentrated on Russell's beliefs concerning good and bad medicine.

When I first arrived at Russell Willier's place to do field-work I noticed that at night before going to bed he would walk around the house holding a smouldering piece of fungus. He would stop and carefully wave the burning incense around the edges of all the windows and doors in the house, praying in Cree. When I asked about the purpose of his behaviour Russell explained that he was 'smoking the windows' because he had recently had a run of bad luck connected with one of his former patients, whom I will refer to as Joe.

Russell had treated Joe four years earlier for a back problem, and Joe had gotten better. Recently, however, he had become seriously ill. Joe had gone to a few other medicine men for help without improving before coming to see Russell once more. Russell took one look at him and knew that Joe was suffering from a curse and that 'the curse was too strong.' Russell could be of no help at this stage. Joe could barely walk and would periodically swell up in different parts of his body. Russell knew of a medicine man in Montana who could possibly deal with such a severe case.

Russell accompanied Joe to Montana, where Joe received two days of sweats and treatment from the other medicine man. He appeared to get better, but at a specific point in the return trip he felt something 'hit.' His condition worsened.

Russell drove Joe down to Montana a second time for further treatment. Again, Joe appeared to get better. On arriving home Joe said that he had a small headache at the back of his neck, but otherwise felt fine. Russell left some tea with him that had been prepared by the medicine man from Montana. Two hours later Russell received a telephone call from Joe's relatives informing him that Joe had been taken to the hospital with a brain haemorrhage. Joe died in the hospital. Russell concluded that the curse had 'worked its way up' from Joe's back, eventually leading to the brain haemorrhage.

Russell then received word from the Montana medicine man warning him of the possibility that a curse had been directed his way. According to Russell, a bad medicine man lives near the spot where Joe was stricken on the return trip from Montana. This medicine man spends his time travelling around and hiring himself out to people who want to have curses sent. Although he doesn't heal, he has the backing of seven legitimate medicine men whom he has deceived. After Joe had been cursed, Russell took him to Montana to get the curse reversed, but the bad medicine man proved too strong. So the curse was sent back to

Joe once again, this time killing him. Because Russell was responsible for taking Joe to Montana, thus allying himself with the Montana healer, he and his family were in danger of being cursed by the bad medicine man. In response, Russell established an invisible circle of power around the entire house and carefully purified the inside of the house each night.

When Russell was a young man starting out on the healing road he visited a medicine man who he thought could help him gain knowledge about his newly-acquired medicine bundle. The medicine man mistakenly believed Russell had come to enlist his services in order to send a curse. The man brought Russell inside his house where he had a cloth tied in a bundle. When he opened the bundle, Russell saw many different kinds of herbs inside. The medicine man told Russell, 'My boy, what you see represents the best of my knowledge. I can send these out anytime you want, anywhere you want.' The medicine man then produced a strangely speckled rock, which Russell surmised was a radioactive substance like uranium. The medicine man waved this rock about a foot over the top of the herbs. The herbs lifted up and hovered above the cloth. Russell explains that the herbs were 'waiting' to go at the medicine man's command. If Russell had actually come to this person to hire his services as a bad medicine man it would have cost from two to four thousand dollars, depending on the kind of curse sought.

Russell explained another form of curse that bad medicine men use, one that does not necessitate the use of herbs. This involves what is called a spiritual attack. A bad medicine man enlists the help of the bad spirits to carry out a curse. Russell explained that sometimes the victim of a curse will glimpse a shadowy figure out of the corner of his or her eye. When spotted the figure disappears immediately. It is what Russell refers to as a shadow spirit. A shadow spirit is instructed to stay close to the intended victim until the moment when the person is at his or her most vulnerable. The shadow spirit may be instructed to attack, for example, when the person is drunk. The bad medicine man knows a victim's vulnerabilities in advance and instructs the bad spirit accordingly.

To break a person financially, a bad medicine man may use herbs ground up into a fine powder and spread on the ground inside a marked-out area. A ritual is performed, and the powdered herbs dematerialize, travelling unseen through the air to hit the victim. One result of such a curse is that others will regard the victim in a negative light. The victim will come to be ignored or disliked. People will see only the bad side of this person, and even the person's family and best friends will reject him or her. In this way the victim is on the way to social and financial ruin.

Curses can also be directed by a bad medicine man through certain animals and through birds like owls or woodpeckers. If a woodpecker pecks on one's house, precautions must be taken against a curse. No matter how the curse is sent, the resulting misfortune appears to everyone else as bad luck, an accident, or the victim's own doing.

The threat of being cursed has been important in Russell's life and work. He has managed to avoid bad medicine men and attempts to inflict misfortune on him, but it has been a struggle. The early years of his career as a healer can be seen as a constant battle against malevolent forces. The period from 1980 to 1985 was the most difficult for Russell, but at the time of the fieldwork he believed that bad medicine men were 'easing off.' They were not attempting to send many curses his way because Russell had been able to withstand them. 'I stood my ground,' he said. 'They don't try much anymore.' Recent events, however, including the death of his father, may have changed his opinion.

In 1987 his father died of a heart attack while Russell was in Edmonton. Soon afterwards his mother was involved in a car accident, sustaining injuries that led to serious complications. A series of such events resulted in what might be termed a life crisis. This was eased only by the rattle ceremony described in the previous chapter.

Prior to the rattle ceremony, Russell described what was happening as a 'hell of a war.' There were various people, he believed, who hired the services of different bad medicine men to direct curses against himself and his relatives. Two of Russell's brothers lost important political positions as a result of bad medicine that caused them to be perceived in a negative light. An office building being built by the Willier family in a nearby town was halted in mid-construction and tied up with a variety of liens. This was done by way of bad medicine, 'out of pure jealousy,' according to Russell.

Russell's father had been in good health. One day he experienced a pain resembling a needle being stuck into his shoulder joint. This occurred several days before his heart attack. A week previously, Russell's mother had experienced a similar needle-like pain in her thigh. Russell doctored his mother successfully. Russell believes the pain was transferred from his mother to the shoulder of his father. The sharp pain moved to various points in his father's body, with the result that he was unable to sleep at night. Russell administered the same medicinal combination to his father as he had used successfully with his mother. His father felt well again after drinking the herbal tea.

On the day that Russell left for Edmonton he visited with his father until after lunch. His father was joking and feeling fine. Russell thought he had removed the effects of the curse. While in Edmonton, Russell received a phone call telling him that his father had been outside walking when he suddenly dropped dead. Russell believes that the curse, which was probably herbal in origin, was only dormant after treatment. The next attack hit his father's heart. Not content with the death of Russell's father, the bad medicine man again attacked Russell's mother, causing her to become involved in a car accident. She was assisted in the hospital by spirits contacted during the rattle ceremony and eventually regained her health.

Russell knows who is responsible for the curses. This person paid a lot of money to hit Russell and his family. The bad medicine man who sent the fatal curse to Russell's father is the same person who sent the curse that killed Joe. He has been kept informed of the activities of Russell and his family by the person who hired his services. Other bad medicine men are out to harm Russell, but this one is the most powerful. Russell meditated and consulted the good spirits to determine the identity of the bad medicine man. Russell says that he was able to see this person's spirit, and it 'was pure evil.'

CONVERSATIONS

The subject of cursing was brought up in the course of a late-night journey to Dawson Creek, British Columbia, to answer an emergency call. Russell and I were travelling down a deserted highway, and the stars were bright above us in the summer sky. On one side of the road we saw the shimmering lights of a town, on the other side the scattered lights of a small settlement.

The conversation began with Russell indicating the lights off in the distance. He asked me to put myself in the place of a bad medicine man.

'If the reflections in the night sky were to represent the medicine circles of two different healers, and your intention were to inflict a curse, which medicine man would you choose to attack?'

'I'd probably attack there,' I said, indicating the settlement.

'This is what I'm trying to tell you. When the medicine men look through someone, this is what they see. They see how strong the medicine man is. Now if a medicine man looked like that [indicating the town], not too many guys would attack him. And that's how people's lights look if you were to go up in the sky and look down.'

'Would a bad medicine man have a light like that, too?'

'Yes. It wouldn't be the same, but it would be similar. You could see how powerful he is.'

'But how would you know it was a bad medicine man from looking at it?'

'Hmm ... well, it's pretty hard for me to answer that question, because I don't mess around with bad medicine. But what I'm trying to tell you is that this is how a bad medicine man sees you. This is how they look at you. If they see you have a light like that [indicating the small settlement], they would try to get rid of you, wipe you out. That's what I've been trying to tell you. The doctoring is not that bad; it's surviving that's tough.'

'You were saying that the attacks have stopped now because the bad medicine men might think you've reached a certain level. But what happens when you go beyond that level?'

'It's hard to say. They don't want you to be big. They don't want you to be like that [indicating the town], ever, because then they couldn't touch you.'

'What would a light look like that was unpredictable?'

'Sometimes the light'll come up and go back out. From the stories that are circulating, they don't really know if you're on the good side or the bad side. That way you keep them hopping. They don't know if they should attack or not.'

'But at a certain point, the good spirits would be more powerful than the bad ones, eh?'

'Yeah. Well, there was one Bible story about the man Job. He had a family, ten or twelve kids. He had everything. Then he came down with some kind of disease. God was checking his faith. Took all of his children away from him. He was down and out and next to nothing. All his friends came over and told him that maybe he's in the wrong religion. But he kept his faith that there's a Great Spirit. He stuck with it. He didn't back off. If you look at it the Indian way, we would say he was cursed. He was overpowered by bad medicine and that's why he lost out. He was crippled. He had no kids. He had nothing, the old guy. He was challenged and he was beaten. Then he came back. He got back to just about where he was before. He got kids and everything, and then he died, according to that story. You see, the way we would look at it, he got beat by bad medicine. Even though he was on the right track, he got wiped out.'

'Once you lose your ability to heal by sending a curse, can you get it back again?'

'No, you can't do that.'

'Even if you completely changed?'

'You never know, because spirits have kind hearts.'

'But could a bad medicine man become a good medicine man?'

'Most people try to change after they get so far. But if you practice bad medicine so far, when you get so wicked, as soon as you stop you're going to die.'

'I see. But if you're only into it so far is there still a chance?'

'It's hard for me to say because I was never on that road. But somebody that's already into bad medicine, if they try to stop, they'll have no power. So what's going to happen? It's going to hit them. They're going to be six feet in the ground.' Here Russell paused for a long time. 'That's why I say that as long as they're active they've pretty well got to keep on. They had a choice when they first started. But it's the greed and jealousy that gets them. Any man, not only the Indian.'

Russell believes there exists a network of bad medicine men across North America who continually watch each other, as well as all those who heal. The moment one achieves success, or 'sticks up too far,' curses will be activated to bring the person down again, 'to level him.' In order to survive, a medicine man that has left the good road has to attract followers. A bad medicine man creates the illusion of having the ability to heal, thus building a clientele. This is done to protect oneself from other bad medicine men and to prevent bad medicine from being returned. The followers act as unknowing shields, as in the case of a girl who was inadvertently killed by a deflected curse. Only through consolidating a group of followers is a bad medicine man able to insulate himself from his own and other bad medicine.

Both healing power and bad medicine are linked with the ability to alter the colours of light that people emit. Everyone has a spirit manifested in light. For healing purposes this light can be controlled in the sweat-lodge. Russell gives 'protectors' to his patients to ensure that a bad medicine man will not be able to change their light and break their medicine circle. A protector is usually a small pouch containing various objects of power. Bad medicine men distribute protectors to their followers in order to deceive them into feeling secure. These protectors, however, change the followers' lights, so that they may become vulnerable to curses being returned by a good medicine man, allowing the bad medicine man to go unscathed.

Returning a curse has unpredictable consequences. If the bad medicine man responsible for the curse is more powerful than a good medicine man who attempts to return it, there is a chance

that the curse will be deflected back to the good medicine man
and cause misfortune. If the curse is successfully returned by a
sufficiently powerful, good medicine man, it could injure or kill
the bad medicine man or any of the followers. Thus, a good
medicine man does not return a curse unless it is absolutely
necessary.

Some of the most interesting conversations about Russell's
concept of bad medicine began around the kitchen table after
the rest of the family had gone to bed. The following conversation occurred when I was just beginning to understand cursing.

'You mentioned that bad medicine men have followers. Are
they like apprentices to the bad medicine man?'

'No. A follower is somebody that comes to you and has a sort
of faith in you. They ask things of you. You give them something
to gain an extra follower. Bad medicine men will hit that person
before they'll hit you.'

'I don't understand.'

'All right. Let's just say you've got to be concerned about
yourself. Some people start coming to you from different places.
So you give all these guys phoney protectors, okay?'

'What is a protector?'

'A protector is something that keeps the bad guys from changing your light. What it does is to make sure that your light does
not change, even if somebody sends something to you. Let's say
he gives all these guys protectors. But sometimes he'll send
something out like bad medicine. If it's returned, it can land on
any one of the followers by mistake.'

'But I still don't understand what a protector is. How does
that work?'

'A protector is something that will be given to you, and you
possess it all the time.'

'Can you see it? Can you see a protector?'

'Yes. You'll have it in a little pouch, which you keep with you.
You will be told to make sure that you put it away when the
women have their monthlies. There are certain things that you
have to do to it. You smoke it, this and that. A protector will
help you. The good guys and the bad guys have protectors. Now

let's say you went to a bad guy and asked for a protector so no one can change your light. This guy then sends some of his bad stuff out to curse someone, to cause a heart attack, or to break them financially, okay? But the guy that gets jinxed turns around and goes to see a good medicine man. The good medicine man takes the curse off and sends it back. He tries to send it back to the bad medicine man, the guy who sent it in the first place. But the bad medicine man is protected by all these little followers. So often it will not land on the bad medicine man. Good medicine men do good, so if good luck returns their followers should be lucky. When bad medicine men have a curse returned their followers will have bad luck.'

LIFTING A CURSE

Russell's method of lifting a curse can be illustrated by an event that took place when Russell's family was visiting the home of David Young. Russell's daughter, Amy, four years old at the time, had arisen one morning with a stomach-ache. She had had a similar stomach-ache on the four previous mornings. Because the pain occurred at the same time each day, Russell decided the stomach-ache was the result of a curse. He pulled up Amy's shirt and marked a circle on her stomach with the burnt end of a fungus incense stick. He formed a second circle inside the charcoal-coloured one, this time using a special herb that he got from a jar. He rubbed the marked-out area with tobacco, praying the whole while. Russell then placed his mouth on Amy's stomach and blew hard four times. After that, he said the stomach-ache would probably not return. But if the pain persisted, he would have to resort to returning the curse to its sender, in which case it would go back four times as strong. It might even be strong enough to kill the person responsible. Asked if he had to know who the sender was in order to return the curse, Russell said this information was not necessary, as the spirits would automatically know, though he could guess who the sender was. Amy appeared to be frightened by the procedure and was relieved when Russell finished.

The stomach-ache did not return.

Russell will avoid returning a curse if at all possible. Twice, David Young observed Russell lifting a curse, which is different from returning a curse. The first occasion was when David Young travelled with Russell to a small Dogrib Indian settlement in the Northwest Territories. Russell had made an earlier trip to the village. He had been invited by the resident medical doctor to visit the settlement in order to demonstrate the Cree use of the sweat-lodge. It is traditional for a medicine man entering another healer's territory to pay that person a visit in order to receive permission to do any doctoring. Russell was not aware at the time of his first visit of a ninety-seven-year-old shaman living in the settlement. The old man knew in advance that another medicine man was approaching. He 'spirit-travelled' to a river crossing marking the entrance to his area in order to check on Russell. When the old man arrived at the river Russell was camped in a nearby clearing. The old man was pleased with what he found. Russell later learned about the shaman from the medical doctor who had invited him to visit. When the old man met Russell he told of his visit and described Russell's camp in detail. Russell was impressed, and the two became good friends.

On the second visit with David Young, Russell visited the old shaman soon after his arrival. Later that day Russell was summoned to treat a person who believed he was being cursed. This person was a productive member of the community who had been experiencing anxiety severe enough to prevent him from going about his usual activities. When Russell and David visited this person's house, David asked if he knew who was responsible for sending the curse. The man named the old shaman Russell had just been to see. This put Russell in a bind. The man wanted the curse to be sent back, but Russell did not believe the old shaman had sent the curse, because in Russell's opinion 'the old man is not on the bad side.' To resolve the situation Russell performed a ceremony to lift – rather than return – the curse. A curse presumably cannot be returned to an innocent individual. Lifting the curse avoided a debate about the identity of the sender and thereby took Russell off the hook. To have the curse lifted, the man was instructed to stand on a cloth print while Russell sprinkled tobacco around him. Russell chewed a herb that filled the room with its fragrant scent. With the herb in his mouth Russell then blew sharply on the person, directing his exhalations to the top of the person's head and to points on each side of the head and neck. Russell rubbed the patient down both sides of his body, pushing the curse off the patient's feet into the tobacco on the print. Russell tied the tobacco up in the print and took it home to be buried or burned.

Russell thinks the reason some people consider the old shaman to be a bad medicine man is that some of his relatives may have asked him to intervene spirtually for them in court appearances. When someone is thought to be guilty of a crime and is not punished resentments build up. Accusations of bad medicine often begin in this manner. It is difficult in native society to refuse a relative's request, even though you might suspect that the person is guilty. Technically, this is an inappropriate use of medicine.

On the same trip to the Northwest Territories, the father-in-law of the man who had the curse lifted suffered from persistent headaches. He believed that he too had been cursed by the old shaman and asked Russell for help. When entering the man's house for the first time Russell had the impression that something was wrong. He felt the house was somehow unhealthy. He prayed, asking the Great Spirit to remove the curse from the house, and purified the place with a burning piece of fungus.

Russell did not believe that the father-in-law himself was cursed, so he did not perform a curse-lifting ceremony. Instead, he ground up several herbs he uses to treat headaches, placed the powder on a red-hot rock, and asked the man to bend over it and inhale deeply while blankets were placed over his head. Russell entered a trance and communed with the spirit world. After about ten minutes the blankets were removed and Russell announced that he had received a communication from the spirit world. He asked the man if he wore glasses. The man said he should be wearing glasses, as his eyesight was poor, but the prescription glasses he had gotten in Yellowknife were not right, because there was a language barrier between himself and the eye doctor. He had thrown away the prescription glasses and purchased a cheap pair for reading. Russell said the spirits had told him that these cheap glasses were the cause of the headaches. Russell told the son-in-law, who spoke good English, to go back to the doctor with his father-in-law and act as a translator so that a good pair of glasses could be obtained.

In Russell's struggle to avoid curses, he learned from another medicine man how to act in a way that makes it difficult for bad medicine men to attack him. Russell calls it 'being unpredictable.' This means that Russell keeps bad medicine men guessing as to what road he is on. Bad medicine men would have to study the situation before directing a curse at Russell, uncertain as to whether or not he might retaliate. Russell initiated a great variety of unrelated projects while I was doing field-work – part of his technique for preventing bad medicine men from knowing in what direction a curse could be effectively placed.

Russell believes that there are two ways of becoming immune to bad medicine. The attainment of a large sum of money, about two million dollars, is one way. This is difficult to achieve for a native person, and few have actually become immune to cursing in this way. 'Going far enough in your medicine' is another way to become invulnerable to curses. These two routes are not contradictory, as they both involve gaining a degree of power that would be impossible to attain without assistance from the spirit world. Thus, great economic and medicine power are signs that one is on the right road and is 'a force to be reckoned with.' Those with power are above the constant warfare among medicine men.

Russell wants to gain sufficient spiritual power so as not to be bothered by bad medicine. This involves attaining the shaking tipi. It is a difficult and risky quest, but the benefits are considerable. A person must be committed and his or her heart must be in the right place in order to succeed.

If Russell Willier is able to attain the shaking tipi, he will be well on his way to achieving access to power. When a bad medicine man directs a curse at Russell or someone he is doctoring, all Russell can do at present is to neutralize or return it. A person with the shaking tipi has more options. Such a person is able to do anything he wants with a curse and also gain new kinds of knowledge. Russell would be able to know in advance if someone is coming to see him for healing, what time the person is arriving, and the nature of the ailment. He would know everything he needed to know about that person. With access to such powers, Russell would become immune to bad medicine. As Russell says, 'If I attain the shaking tipi, no one will be able to touch me.'

But what has cursing to do with healing? To answer this, we must return once more to the question of what a curse is. It might seem that Russell is not interested in what Western medicine calls the etiology of disease. This is not true. Russell is aware of what we would call pathological processes involving germs or viruses, but he believes that illness cannot be understood by reference to these alone. The pathological processes themselves may be the result of bad medicine.

The important issue has to do with why certain people attract curses. The answer is a moral one. People who attract curses are those who have violated their society's ethical code. By being greedy, selfish, envious, and 'sticking out too far,' such people get out of balance with themselves and their community. They suffer guilt and attract misfortune carried by a curse. The healer restores balance. This is accomplished by a series of rituals involving, among other things, counselling, prayer, and chanting, all of which may be incorporated into the sweat-lodge, rattle, and pipe ceremonies.

Generally, anthropologists and other social scientists view witchcraft and sorcery as mechanisms of social control, levelling devices whose sociological function is to keep people from breaking established rules. According to this 'functional approach,' witchcraft and sorcery also have the psychological function of displacing emotional frustrations that build up as a result of day-to-day conflicts. These sociological and psychological functions of witchcraft and sorcery are frequently regarded by functionalists as being beneficial, or positive, though the potential for social disruption is recognized.

The functional approach perceives social phenomena like witchcraft and sorcery as exerting influences beyond the awareness of individuals. The 'function' of what individuals do is seen as an unintended consequence of their combined actions. The problem with functionalism is that it either ignores or does not take seriously people's own views of what is happening and what should happen in society.

It is our position that to understand social life it is not necessary to consider people's views as irrational and their actions as under the sway of functional influences. Russell Willier is aware of the functionalist perspective on witchcraft and sorcery. He has developed a model emphasizing that cursing is an explicit levelling device designed to increase conformity to society. Unlike functionalists, however, Russell does not see this as beneficial. He believes that the disruptive effects of cursing on individual's lives must be countered by the balancing, healing rituals of the good medicine man.

I have avoided the question of whether curses and bad medicine actually have the power to influence events – whether they 'work.' Some researchers have dealt with this by suggesting the influence of psychological factors in the case of a person who has been a victim of so-called bad medicine. Someone who dies as a result of bad medicine is said to have been so stricken by fear that the nervous system went into a fatal state of shock, and there are well-documented cases of this. This sort of explanation does not accord with Russell's view that curses are effective whether or not people know they have been cursed.

There is much that scientific knowledge cannot at present account for in the healing process. For example, the Chinese are doing a good deal of experimentation with 'Qi,' translated roughly as vital force. Qi-Gong masters train for years to build up and project externally this force that is believed to reside in all things. Practitioners have demonstrated their ability to effect change in both animate and seemingly inanimate objects. Demonstrations have shown that Qi-Gong masters are able to move objects without touching them, stimulate movement in paralysed patients, and alter bacterial growth patterns under laboratory conditions. There is lethal Qi and health-promoting Qi.

The concept of Qi seems alien to someone from a Western culture, and its effects have not yet been measured or systematically documented. The Chinese are currently engaged in cooperative research with other countries to attempt to measure Qi force through such sophisticated instruments as nuclear magnetic resonance scanners, computed tomography (CT) scanners, and other electromagnetic devices. Such research is motivated by the belief that phenomena we do not at present understand should not be arbitrarily dismissed as solely the result of the power of suggestion.

Many levels of reality coexist within the natural world, levels that modern science has only begun to explore. If life is viewed in these terms it is not necessary to conceive of mutually exclusive orders of things. Distinctions between the natural and supernatural realms and between religious and scientific phenomena are beginning to break down. Unexplained things, including the effects of cursing, may have a material basis. Until this basis is better understood, we must proceed on the assumption that the curse, however it is understood, is a vital, lethal force that must be counteracted by Russell Willier as he seeks to protect himself, his relatives, and his followers, and to restore his patients to good health and fortune.

❡ Nature's Medicine Cabinet

Russell Willier, who has always felt a special affinity with nature, is well versed in the uses of roots, barks, and leaves that can be combined into effective medicines based on formulas passed down through generations of his Woods Cree ancestors. His healing remedies are collected from the forests, fields, and lakes in northern Alberta. Concerned that much of this knowledge will disappear, Russell decided to show us some of the plants that are available for use as medicines, with the hope that together we might find a way of protecting and preserving the plants and plant lore for future generations.

One day in mid-June 1985 we travelled to the Lesser Slave Lake area to go on a botanical field trip with Russell. This area of Alberta's boreal forest contains varying combinations of deciduous poplar, spruce, jack-pine, birch, aspen, balsam fir, and tamarack. The undergrowth is very lush and rich in species of plants and animals. There is a profusion of ponds, sloughs, willow swamps, reed marshes, and muskegs.

The following day we walked with Russell through the woods at the western shores of Lesser Slave Lake, and Russell pointed out the various plants and trees he uses in his doctoring. He explained to us that 'if you put tobacco on the first plant taken then you're going to see that kind of plant all over'. He knelt before a plant, prayed in Cree, and placed a small handful of tobacco in the ground. He was now allowed to take some of the plants of that species for medicine.

As we walked along Russell explained that the samples of young trees and saplings that are necessary for his combinations are taken from the plant just above the root at ground level. A portion the width of one's hand is taken from the main stem, the top of which is replanted together with an offering of tobacco. Bark collected from a tree or bush – aspen, poplar, saskatoon, or choke-cherry – is taken from the east or south sides. Periodically, when Russell was reluctant to disclose the specific use of a plant, he would simply tell us that 'it goes in a combination.' Walking along the road back to our camp, Russell informed us that the different colours of flowers represent the different parts of the sacred circle. Yellow stands for east, blue represents west, white is north, and red is south.

'What is herbal doctoring?' one of us inquired.

'Herbal doctoring is where we take the plants that God has put upon this earth for mankind to use. All the plants and trees and animals have got something that they can give to help cure different sicknesses. If you get herbs from Mother Earth and if you make an offering, for example putting down tobacco, or you promise things to Mother Nature, such as fasting for three or four days, it's repaid back slowly in that the herbs can be used in doctoring and they're effective. Nature is sacred; the herbs, they are very holy. God, the Great Spirit, put them there a long time ago, long before the Bible was written. Herbal doctoring is all around the world, and as a matter of fact it probably existed in Jerusalem in the day of Moses. They were probably doing some herb doctoring. It's not written in the Bible, but how else would they be doctoring? God probably told them about which plants they could put together in combinations. That's why the ancient Hebrews were so holy that they could perform miracles; they were getting their power right from nature. That's where the power is. That's where most people in the different churches misinterpret the power and communion of God. They forget about nature.'

'Would you say that almost every kind of animal and plant has some use?'

'Yes, if a person gets to know nature they could learn much. Most people don't check why that plant or animal is on this earth, how they live, how they breathe, what their purpose is. If you think about the Arctic, for example, look how many animals and plants there are there. What is their purpose? We don't know because it's not Cree territory, but the Inuit probably knows. The same is true for Africa and all the other countries of the world. The animals and plants are there to be used for medicines, and each has a spirit.'

'What happens when a new, unknown disease appears? Will a new plant come into being that has never existed before?'

'It is probably the case that this plant has been waiting to be used. God looks ahead, and that plant could have been waiting all these centuries. But sometimes if you don't use certain plants, God will take them away. The problem now is that there aren't enough medicine men practising who have the knowledge to use all these plants.

'I have tried to transplant certain herbs that are scarce onto my property on the reserve in order to protect them, but you can't always do that since you need the same conditions that they naturally grow in, and I might not have that. Several years ago I transplanted seneca root and small-arrow on my land with the hope that they would grow, but they didn't. Just recently I brought in and planted half an acre of sage, which would save me from driving hundreds of miles to get it, but I don't know yet if it will grow right. It's actually easier to move animals from one area to another than it is to transplant herbs and plants.

'I think man has the capability to transplant animals. We don't have any skunks up north, and they're useless in Edmonton where you find quite a few. Some should be transferred up north. So wherever animals are getting fewer they could be transferred. This makes sense if you look at the environment as a whole. In Saskatchewan they've been moving marten. Some trappers from Saskatchewan asked me for live marten so they can raise them there, which shows that they're also concerned about the lack of certain animals in their forests.'

'If you transferred an animal couldn't you throw nature off balance? For example, if someone brought down a few wolves from northern Alberta wouldn't that change things?'

'It is dangerous for humans to mess around with the balance of nature to a certain extent. But that's why we've got a mind of our own; to use our common sense. Like that man that wanted to raise marten in northern Saskatchewan thought it wouldn't affect the other fur-bearing animals. Maybe the squirrels, but he figured the marten would survive good there. If he let them go for four years on his trapline he could probably earn a few thousand dollars. He asked me to bring four pair of live marten, but I can't do that since I could lose my trapline. Fish and Wildlife officers won't allow transfer of the animals across the border. But people have to understand that the natives still use the animals and the plants in order to get their medicine from them.'

'The tobacco you placed in the ground today when you took some plants, that was for the spirit of the plant? What if you didn't have any tobacco?'

'You're dealing with nature, and the trees and all the herbs are alive and you have to have respect for them, especially when you're taking the herbs or the roots. When we walked through the woods today, to some people it would just be like another day's hiking, but you were getting introduced to different plants all along as we were going through. Usually when we get any kind of herbs from the earth, Mother Earth, or from the water, we always place an offering of tobacco in the ground or water. For example, if you were to pick twelve herbs of the same kind that you needed in a combination, you would take one here and you'd sort of follow the sun, go in a clockwise direction, pick the rest, and come back to where you started. You wouldn't pick one here, pick one over there, pick another here. You don't just grab them from anywhere,' he laughed. 'If you were to pick different herbs, then you would have to put tobacco on each kind that you want and pray,' he emphasized. 'You don't just offer tobacco and hope for the best. The plants that I took today, without putting tobacco down, they're no good for medicine. Just the herbs that I took where I offered tobacco and prayed can be used for doctoring.

'The Crees up here, when they didn't have tobacco, used to use red willow shavings, and that represented tobacco. They gave that as an offering and they made it into tobacco. The whole idea of giving it back to Mother Earth is that you have to open up, get in a state of mind where you'll be talking with or getting help from the spiritual world. The main power from God is right there. You have to be humble, you have to get off your high horse and realize that the blade of grass is worth more than you are. You have to have an open mind.'

'Russell, you mentioned that your great-grandfather passed his medicine bundle over to you and that it contained herbal combinations. When did you inherit this bundle?'

'I got it when I was about seventeen or eighteen years old, but at the time I was just getting into life so I just sort of put it aside; I didn't want to use it because it's something that's sacred. There are two kinds of bundles among the Cree; one has herbs in it and another, the spiritual bundle, would have things like rattles, pipes, a bear claw or porcupine hide in it. Medicine bundles are very powerful. In the past they sometimes buried them in the forests until the right person came along and was recognized as being the right kind of person to get that bundle. He would find it.'

'What about the bundles that are on display in museums. Do they still have power?'

'Some may, but they probably have to awakened. You can't sell a medicine bundle, so if it was sold rather than given to the museum, you would have to awaken it. If you did the proper ritual, like smoke it over sweetgrass or sage and pray, then you should be able to bring the power back to some of these bundles.

'When I started to use my medicine bundle, I had to get the elders to tell me what the herbs were. Bunches of herbs were tied together in the bundle to show the different combinations, but you still had to learn the identity of each herb. I approached the elders to find out what the herbs were and where to find them. I would make a deal with an elder where I'd give him tobacco or a gift and he would show me what the plant looks like when it's in bloom, and the area where it grows, either a swampy area or a dry hill, or sometimes in the water. So you know you can always get that herb from Mother Earth because you've learned what it looks like and where to find it. Once you know the combination, what to put together, it's not that hard.'

'What exactly is a combination, Russell?'

'A combination consists of herbs that are selected and prepared as medicine. Sometimes you only combine a few herbs, but other combinations may require quite a number of herbs and perhaps an animal part as well. I learned some of my combinations from the medicine bundle. The herbs that were tied together to show the combinations were very old. I didn't actually use those herbs but just looked at them to know what they are, and then I got fresh, new herbs from the ground. Other combinations I have learned from elders who have passed them over to me, but sometimes they're hard to get because they don't want to pass combinations over and often you either have to give a four-legged animal or pay a heavy price. You don't just get it; you have to earn it. You have to earn the trust, the love from them, and they can refuse you any time.'

'Would this be the way a medicine man would have learned in the old days, or would he have learned just from one person?'

'I would think if the tribes were moving about, a young man practising medicine would probably hear about certain combinations and treatments from other people or other tribes of Crees. I would think it was the same way as I'm going now.'

'Will the medicine bundle that you will pass on to your son or grandson be bigger than the one that you inherited from your great-grandfather?'

'Yes, I'd say the majority of the medicine bundles that will be passed on will be a lot bigger than they normally would because today we can write the combinations down.'

'So you feel that you will know more and have a greater variety of herbs to use than people did fifty or sixty years ago?'

'No, I think what happened is they kept the best combinations, the strongest ones. If one were trying to learn about curing earaches or toothaches, they didn't really bother with passing that on. They only passed over the combinations that dealt with the major illnesses, those that meant life or death.'

'Can you tell us a little bit about how you go about getting your herbs? Do you usually collect them in the spring, or does it make any difference what time of year you get them?'

'We usually harvest them in August and the first part of September when they deflower, and then we keep them over the winter. But if somebody wanted to see them, it's better to go when they're flowering. That way you'll know what the herb is. If you saw them in September, well, usually only a medicine man will recognize the plant. He'll know what he's looking for. Even if he lost his vision, then he still has his senses of taste, touch, and smell to know the herb. It is very important for the medicine man to master these senses. He has to know what the herb feels like, how it tastes and smells, and what it looks like in the different seasons.'

'How many different kinds of herbs would you say you work with? Hundreds?'

'No, I watch the combinations very closely, and you actually don't use more than roughly forty herbs altogether. Some combinations may require eight herbs, others twelve. The combinations are the ones that you have to be master of, because if you made something for a patient and his body rejected it, you could poison him. You have to know your herbs in order to put the combination together. Once you get the combination you pretty well have it for the rest of your life until you pass it over to somebody else. And the ones that have been lost, if the medicine man didn't pass them over to someone before he died, they can sometimes be given back by the spiritual world. For example, the spirits might give back a combination to someone by telling them about it in a dream.'

Russell then told us that dreams are very important in connection with herbs. The following story illustrates how he will sometimes gain information through dreams.

One day an older man came to Russell's house to be cured of something. As he didn't have a herb he needed in the house, Russell went out to an old building where he keeps herbs. He knew there were some in a cupboard in the old building, but he couldn't find them. So he told the old man he would be gone for half an hour while he looked for the herb. He jumped in his car and went to a woods where he knew some of the herbs were growing. To his dismay, he looked for an hour without finding any. Finally, discouraged, he sat down to meditate and left a little tobacco as an offering.

Looking over his shoulder, he saw the herb growing right behind him. That night he dreamed about the incident. In his vision a little man about four feet tall came to him. He was the spirit of the herb Russell had been looking for. The little man explained that he had played tricks on Russell, preventing him from finding the herb in the cupboard or in the woods. This was to demonstrate to Russell that he must depend on assistance from the spirits. Then the man told Russell to follow him. He guided him to a beautiful spot in the forest that Russell had never seen. There were trees, a little meadow with that herb growing all over the place, and a path. There were also several elk resting in the meadow.

Later, Russell went elk hunting with one of his friends. His friend took him to the same spot Russell had seen in his dream. Russell told his friend he knew this place and that there should be a little path leading to a meadow where elk would be resting. Russell quickly found the path. Following the path, they came upon the elk and shot two of them. Russell saw a lot of the herb growing there but he did not pick any.

Russell allowed us to help him collect a plant he was running out of one day. I had not realized how much work was involved. After Russell taught us to distinguish the roots of this plant from a poisonous one that looked very similar, we dispersed into the woods to collect, some in pairs, others alone. Russell needed only the root, so he had instructed us to bury the stalk and flowering part of the plant. Since the plant was fairly tall and large, this was an awkward and time-consuming activity.

When we periodically met up with other groups or individuals and compared how many roots we had collected, a kind of playful competition arose to see who could gather the most roots in the shortest time. At one point Grant and Lise decided to combine collections. On transferring Grant's roots to Lise's bag it was noticed that the two collections did not appear to be the same. One of us had, for several hours, been gathering the wrong root. Luckily Judith, an ethnobotanist, was close by and was able to confirm which root was the correct one. This aptly demonstrates the skill required in herb gathering. Many of the plants look very similar in appearance, as do their roots, and it is easy for an amateur to make mistakes. After this experience, I understood why Russell stresses that a medicine man must know the plant through his senses: smell, touch, sight, and taste. If the medicine man were untrained and uncertain about a herb, its use in a combination could be lethal to the patient.

Later in the day, we engaged Russell in a conversation about the use of animals for medicine.

'Russell, you mentioned that you also use animal parts for medicine. Which ones do you use?'

'Yes, we use animals. For example, we use bear, beaver, weasel, wild geese, moose, deer, coyote, horse, and there are some wild ducks that are used for medicine. The bear gall-bladder, for instance, will get rid of a lot of poison. You either drink it or you could use it by rubbing it on, anointing yourself. The way you would use it depends on the illness source. The bear gall-bladder is used by other cultures, too. We received a letter from a Chinese person saying that if I ever had any bear gall-bladders they would be willing to buy them. The bear and the buffalo are used in doctoring patients with back problems, and you can also use one herb we call the backbone herb. All these different animals, and there are lots of them, have a spirit. If you go and get a skunk, you'll ask the Skunk Spirit for help in the cure. These animals, according to our Indian religion, walk on this earth for that purpose. They could be eaten and they could be used for doctoring. A lot of different animals are on this earth for man to use. Like the wild geese; we use their grease for doctoring.

God has put them here for that purpose. So, if I use the bear, say the gall-bladder, then I'll have to ask the Bear Spirit first. Most people get it all so confused, they figure the Indian is just praying to the animals, but that's not the case.'

Russell explained that the animal spirits reside in their namesakes. Thus, the Buffalo Spirit dwells in every buffalo. Each animal exists in nature specifically for people's needs and may become extinct if no longer used. When there is a decline in a particular animal population it could be the result of abuse or because the animal has never been used for its medicinal properties. This presents a paradox, in that it appears to be a belief that encourages hunting an endangered species in an attempt to discover its medicinal value, thereby hastening the decline of the species. Russell has failed to resolve this paradox for us. In his mind there is no necessary contradiction, as the Great Spirit increases the population of a species if convinced that the animals are being used wisely.

Every creature has certain parts with medicinal properties. When the animal is sacrificed, offerings are consecrated to the spirit of the animal and the special parts are purified and used in curing. Often the purification rites are conducted by elders, who place the heart of the animal in the fire as an offering. As with the herbs, animal parts cannot be used as medicine if prayers and offerings are not made at the time of sacrificing the animal. Russell cannot use any part of an animal if he is uncertain whether the hunter performed the necessary prayers and offerings.

Russell calls upon the spirits of the eagle, buffalo, bear, and wild goose to help effect a cure. He says that no one animal is more sacred than another since they are all represented in the spiritual world. An eagle, for example, is not considered mightier than a little mouse. Human beings cannot control the spirits, but through offerings and purification can seek to gain their influence.

'How does one gain the spirit help of a particular animal?'

'A certain animal will actually come to you. Sometimes you obtain their help if you fast for four days and nights all by yourself. A certain animal will come, and you will either see him or hear him. He'll be there, and you'll know that that's the one that will help you. He'll stick with you for quite a long time, and if you follow the Sweetgrass Trail, he'll be with you all the time. You can't guarantee that he'll stay for the rest of your life, particularly if you happen to switch from the good medicine to the bad medicine.'

Not only is Russell a well-known hunter, but he has an intuitive sense of where the animals are. When he wants a moose or any other animal he gets it. His Indian name, Mehkwasskwan (Red Cloud), means that when a hunter sees red clouds at sunset it is a sign that she or he will get the desired animal.

One afternoon in July, Russell and Grant Ingram had gone hunting for moose in the Spirit River area. Although they fired at a moose, it ran away. Early the next morning, they tried again, but this time Russell used 'moose medicine.' He lighted a piece of fungus, with which he purified the truck inside and around the outside. He then purified his gun. Within minutes the hunters came upon two moose, a large cow and a yearling. These animals did not take flight when they saw the hunters but kept on walking across the road. After shooting them both, Russell commented to Grant, 'See the difference; they weren't even scared of us.' Russell said that the 'moose medicine' had been passed to him from his father. When he first received it, he was uncertain as to whether it was actually working or if he was just having a streak of good luck. Since his hunting is very successful whenever he uses the medicine, he has decided that it works; however, he prefers not to use it unless he has to because it may lead to overkill. When leaving the Spirit River area Russell explained that he would not return to hunt there for a year, to allow time for the animals to return.

When Russell skinned and quartered the moose, he cut the heart out and placed it on a tree above his head, then rubbed the heart downwards in a line to the bottom of the tree and covered it with moss. This was the offering to the Moose Spirit. The very back part of the tail of the moose is thrown away, since there is a belief that if this is eaten all the hunter will see is the rear of the moose as it runs away. On their return to the reserve,

Russell distributed the meat to various relatives, who were requested to give some to the elders and widows.

Often Russell must travel long distances to hunt. Skunks, for example, are rare in the Sucker Creek area, so he has to travel more than a hundred miles to get them. Bears also are becoming more difficult to find because they are being shot by the farmers who produce honey.

According to Russell, 'There would be enough bears if the honey farmers left them alone. Bears are attracted to honey from a distance because of the smell of the honey in the air which they can sense five to eight miles from the boxes. I know of one farmer who killed thirty-two bears in one season. This should not be allowed. He just killed them and left them. He didn't use any of the bear, like the gall-bladder, which is very important in Indian medicine. And the fur was no good because he killed the bears in the middle of the summer. The young Fish and Wildlife officers, who are just beginning their training, could learn a great deal by catching the bears from the farmer's area and bringing them thirty or forty miles away.

'Natives have hunted and eaten from nature as long as they can remember. Nowadays, when fall comes, the hunting season should be watched very closely so that you don't have so many hunters out. A lot of these European hunters have four or five hundred head of cattle, and they're out hunting elk and wild sheep. They're people that are actually raising their own stock to eat or raising it for industry, for the people in other parts of the province. And yet they're out hunting. They should leave the animals to the natives and not hunt them anymore.'

'Why do you guide for some of these hunters?'

'Because I've got a family to support and my income is so low. I have to make ends meet. If I could make money elsewhere I wouldn't guide.

'I figured that by discussing these issues openly, maybe people will have more respect for nature. There's a lot of trees that are coming down, actually for no reason, herbs that are being rooted up for no reason and the ground left bare for pigweed and stuff like that to grow. The main herbs are actually disappearing, slowly but surely. There are some of these plants in the combinations that I won't mention because they'll all be dug out, and there's not that many in the country. You can't very well tell anybody about these plants, because you'll lose them all. Sometimes I have to travel two hundred miles to get a plant. I'm scared to give out knowledge of the plants in case they will be overpicked. They'll be uprooted at the wrong time, whereas most natives will take the roots after the plant deflowers and seeds again. But in the cases that I know of where some of the names were given out, they were uprooted in the spring, they were uprooted before they even flowered, and they were all killed off.

'The ones that are really doing the worst damage are the farmers. The farmers and the loggers are wiping out everything. They should consider a lot of things before they just go out there and clean the whole forest right out. We often have to travel long distances to get certain kinds of herbs because they're either ploughed under or they've drained the water right out. Where the marshes go dry the plants quit growing and the ducks leave the area because there's nothing to eat. I was reading some articles by Ducks Unlimited. I guess they're starting to realize that the marshlands in Alberta are draining and drying up. A lot of the plants are disappearing, too. A lot of the ducks are disappearing because the plants are dying off right around them.

'And if a farmer clears out four sections of land or four quarters like they do in my area, they just wipe out the whole works. Instead of leaving a few herbs here and there, they just clear them right out. Perhaps it could be arranged by the government that so many acres could be put aside in a certain part of the country and just left there so the herbs will slowly keep on growing in their natural habitat.

'The game wardens must also consider what happens when you change the environment. For example, because the wolves use the skidoo trails as highways, they're able to reproduce faster and kill more deer, caribou, and moose. When the snow is not disturbed it's harder for the wolves to get around, and now it's much easier. The environmental experts probably don't realize just how fast these wolves are reproducing because of skidoo trails and old snowploughed roads. Wolves can travel a long way and kill what game they can slaughter as they move along. They're very hard to trap because they're wise animals, and they've learned about snares and traps. Few trappers get them.'

'Don't you believe that wolves eat only the old and sick animals?'

'No, the game wardens should watch them more closely and then they would know. For example, about a quarter mile from my trapping cabin they killed a young bull moose. They had just pulled it down when I drove up. I didn't see them actually kill it, but it was fresh and it hadn't been there two hours before. It had four rips on each side of its body. They gutted it and then they all disappeared into the bush. I looked at it and figured I would put traps up tomorrow morning when the wolves were not there. So, early in the morning, about daybreak, I went over, but there was nothing but the bones and a few hairs here and there. They had eaten everything during the night. They were gone and they never did come back.'

'Do you agree with the way they hunt the wolves in British Columbia, by shooting them from helicopters?'

'No, I wouldn't kill the whole pack. Out of a pack of fifteen I would probably take eight or six and leave the rest, because they need each other to survive and if you kill too many of the hunters then the other ones will probably starve to death because they're also teaching one another. If a group of wolves are running, there will probably be only two or three good hunters and the rest are followers. They're growing up and are learning their skills from the older ones, so it's a very touchy thing when you shoot them. Which ones are you going to kill? Are you going to kill the followers to trim them down, or are you going to kill the hunters? I would hunt the young ones, because the hunters will raise other little ones and they will teach them again. But if you kill the old hunters off, these young ones are not going to know a lot of skills that they were supposed to know, and they might not survive. It's just like a human family. If in a family of ten people the majority of the adults got killed, the younger people might not make it.'

'Can you recognize which ones are the hunters?'
'They should be able to from the air, because the wolves would be running, and the hunters would be ahead, out in front.'

ECOLOGICAL AWARENESS

The nature of the relationship between Indian peoples and the environment has been a much discussed and disputed issue among anthropologists, politicians, and environmentalists. At one extreme, reports of early explorers, traders, missionaries, and other firsthand observers of native societies have led to the allegation that North American Indians irrationally slaughtered wildlife and decimated the buffalo and fur-bearing animals. At the other extreme, Indians have been extolled as 'noble savages' and ecological saints who live in harmony with all creation. This second view helped to elevate the Indian to a position of spiritual leadership in the ecology movement that began in North America in the 1960s. Concerned environmentalists advocated learning from the Indians' understanding of nature to prevent further ecological crises.

Anthropologists with a functional orientation have explained the relationship between native people and land-use as one in which Indian rituals and practices have beneficial ecological consequences (although not necessarily by intention). Other researchers have argued convincingly that Indian people are indeed rational in respect to their environment and that they consciously control their natural resources.

In early accounts by explorers, traders, and missionaries, we find the most damaging stereotyping of the Indian, who is blamed for the extermination of the bison herds. Herds of up to several hundred bison were driven over large cliffs in what is today known as a bison jump. This was done once a year, usually in the fall, in order to obtain enough meat to see the tribes through the long winter when other animals were scarce. The jump technique required a large number of animals in order to be successful. Those in front would be able to see the approaching danger, but it was impossible for them to turn away with the large numbers of bison behind them.

Despite the many animals killed in this type of hunt, it was not wasteful. All parts of the bison were used, for food, clothing, shelter, tools, and ritual objects. Meat was dried to make pemmican, which could be eaten throughout the winter. Moreover, killing a few hundred animals did not deplete the bison population, which at that time was in the millions. The Plains Indians hunted bison for thousands of years without endangering the species. It was only when the Europeans arrived in North America that the bison herds began to disappear and eventually became almost extinct. Guns, horses, and the railroad were major factors contributing to the demise of the bison.

Another myth concerns the fur trade, an event initiated by the arrival of Europeans. The most common explanation for the Indians' participation in the fur trade at the time of contact with Europeans is an economic one. Many fur-bearing animals were trapped and hunted by native people in their attempt to improve their standard of living through trade for European goods and materials. Over-exploitation did not occur prior to contact because there was a limited market for the furs. Moreover, the spiritual relationship between native people and animals prevented overkilling. Along with the privilege of hunting animals, which were expected to give their lives to people for food and clothing, went obligations. Hunters had to show respect for the animal and to perform proper rituals pertaining to the use of the animal; they were not to kill more than they needed and not to torture or abuse the animal in any way.

Long before contact with Europeans, hunting and trapping constituted the way of life for Canadian Indians. In many northern communities today it is still the primary life-style, and values are centred on hunting and trapping activities. But there is tremendous controversy over trapping, and the conservation movement has effectively destroyed whole economies in northern Canada during the last decade. The European boycott of the fur industry does not recognize or acknowledge that hunting and trapping are the lifeblood of these communities.

In May 1988 a native radio program reported on the most recent fight against the fur industry. Animal rights groups in Britain are campaigning very strongly against the fur industry in all its forms, including fur farms and trapping. As a result, the British minister of trade proposed a law that labels must be sewn into fur coats made from furs of animals caught in a leg-hold trap. Animals commonly caught in this manner include several varieties of fox, lynx, bobcat, coyote, and wolf. Although the proposed law was withdrawn, a preliminary survey of the reaction of consumers to the idea indicated that they would avoid purchasing fur coats with such a label and would look for coats made from animals raised on farms. If such a law is ever passed, it would, of course, have disastrous effects on the fur industry and be even more devastating for the native communities that rely on trapping for subsistence.

We have discussed some of the factors giving rise to various stereotypes of North American Indians. Let us now take a closer look at this controversy in relation to where Russell stands with respect to his environment. When doing field-work with some-one like Russell, one finds that none of the above explanations adequately portrays Russell's relationship with the environment. There is concern about protecting nature, but there is also the necessity to obtain one's food and livelihood from the land. It is a matter of striking a balance. Russell told us that he often hauls fish heads and other animal remains to his trapline. By doing this he is both helping preserve the animal populations that need food and helping himself, since there will be more animals available on his trapline.

Russell is aware of the political struggles now occurring over native land-claims issues. But he is also aware of his limited power to affect these larger issues and has a realistic understand-ing of the extent of his influence. He may not be able to effect change in the area of treaty rights and land claims, but he does try to institute changes in less politically explosive areas. Envi-ronmental changes that he suggests are realistic rather than uto-pian. One of Russell's hopes is that this book will be widely read and become a means for increasing public pressure on the gov-ernment to make changes. Every day there are new reports of the environmental damage that occurs across Canada. The general lack of response to these problems demonstrates that environmental issues are not considered political priorities. The time has come when most countries of the world, especially industrialized countries, must confront the consequences of development and economic growth without environmental assessment and planning.

Russell is concerned about regulating changes to undeveloped land at the planning stage, rather than trying to rectify irreparable damage after it is done. If, he suggests, the government intends to lease or sell sections of land to farmers in any one area, or if large areas are destined for clear-cutting for timber, half-mile strips of natural surround should be left. He used the example of Westlock, a small commuity north of Edmonton, to demonstrate the adverse effects when forests and bush are destroyed. The area consists mainly of farmland, and there are miles and miles of fields without any bush, forest, or wilderness. If strips of natural vegetation were left dispersed across such an area, they would not only preserve the herbs and plants but also provide shelter for deer, pheasants, foxes, and other creatures who make their homes in these ecological niches. The strips should be considered as restricted areas and should be left wherever land is being cleared either for farming or logging. These strips should not be limited to any one specific environmental area but should be spread throughout the country.

Road development in northern Alberta inevitably opens up the wilderness for farming and therefore is another area of concern for Russell. First come the paved roads, next poles for electricity, and then the farmers. Within a few years, the former wilderness consists of endless fields. Russell and other medicine men see the grim consequences of continued development of wilderness areas with no consideration for long-term ecological repercussions. But Russell says that their own 'tongues are not powerful enough,' and that change must be effected by those in power. They ask those who have the authority in decision-making when land development is in the planning stage to consider the needs of native people. Many native people rely heavily on wild plants and animals for food and herbal medicine. Leaving strips of wilderness across Canada is necessary for the continuation of traditional native medicine.

When asked if Indian reserves had considered acquiring additional land to enlarge natural habitats for animal populations, Russell explained the complexity of such action. If someone wants to acquire land, the government offers grant money to clear the land. After the land is cleared and used for agricultural purposes for a certain length of time, the settler receives title to the land. Moreover, the government has restricted acquisition of public lands to homesteaders, and since it has stipulated that this land must subsequently be cleared, native reserves do not have the opportunity to extend reserve areas for hunting purposes. If they could, this would of course produce additional livelihood for many native hunters. Russell remembers, when he was growing up, hunting on horseback in the wilderness around the Sucker Creek Reserve. Today, that land is mostly farmland. He believes that in a few years there will be very few animals left for hunting, as the government continues to encourage homesteading in the area.

Russell asked David Young to assist him and a fellow medicine man to get a section of the Swan Hills set aside as a place of religious retreat for native people. This land is in the centre of the area traditionally used by natives for vision-quest purposes. Logging is being done nearby, and Russell is concerned that the vision-quest sites may soon be ruined. Russell would like to continue to have a place to take young people for a wilderness experience that would include instruction in the vision-quest, survival skills, the Sweetgrass Trail, and other traditional native skills and knowledge. He would also like to instil in native young people traditional values connected with hunting, particularly a respect for the animals and a responsiveness to the delicate balance of nature. This means teaching them to exercise control over the numbers of animals killed, to vary the seasons and places in which animals are hunted, and to obey the fishing and hunting regulations.

Russell explained his own special relationship with certain

animals and their spirits. For example, when the Beaver Spirit enters him, he ends up working like a beaver. This special connection, however, does not prevent him from killing the animal when he needs it for food or medicine. There is a difference, in his opinion, between sacrificing an animal for specific needs and needlessly killing animals. He only hunts when he needs the animal for food or medicine. Killing an animal for these reasons does not anger the spirit of the animal. When he hunts successfully he shares the meat with elders and members of his family. One should never hunt out of greed or kill more animals than are absolutely nesessary.

Some hunters kill indiscriminately for their own profit. Russell has suggested to his band council the need to control those who engage in large kills, wasting animals. This could be accomplished by turning them in to the Fish and Wildlife authorities. But bringing irresponsible native hunters to the attention of government officials might jeopardize treaty rights.

It is important that more native people become Fish and Wildlife officers. This would give them the authority to discipline those few who create problems for everyone, and they would likely have a better understanding of native needs and environmental issues. As Russell says, his ancestors have been hunting in this area for many centuries while maintaining long-term ecological balance. Experienced hunters had a vast knowledge of the resources of the land and the changing conditions of game populations. Their hunting practices were characterized by their willingness to exercise self-control. Even today, successful hunters who exhibit competence, skill, and spirituality, and who do not hunt excessively, are respected and are often contrasted with those who hunt recklessly.

Russell sees a great deal of waste of animal remains that could be used to regenerate wildlife. Most big-game hunters dispose of moose remains and other large animal intestines by throwing them in the dump. They should be required to leave the remains behind in the forest or bring them to the trapline where other animals can eat them. This is particularly important for large, commercial fisheries. Although fisheries located on Lesser Slave

Lake are regulated by quotas set by the government, their means of disposal of fish-heads and other remains is not only wasteful but also destroys wildlife. The present practice is to dump the remains in a large hole, which is then covered with lye. An animal that comes along and eats the remains dies of lye poisoning. This, says Russell, is representative of the wrong attitude that many non-natives have developed towards the environment, namely 'grab, make a dollar, and forget about the rest.' Fisheries make considerable profit from their catch, and there are enough fish remains to feed many local animals. Dispersing these remains in areas where animals are starving should be mandatory. This would create jobs for native people in northern Alberta where there is much unemployment.

Natives and hunters are worried about the wild duck and geese populations, which get smaller each year. Farmers are not worried. They want more land for hay, and each year in May and June they burn the stubble of their hayfields around the shores of the lake. May and June are nesting times for wildfowl. Eggs, newly hatched ducks and geese, and other birds are burnt while still in their nests. There must, Russell stresses, be a law against the lake fires during nesting season that destroy millions of eggs. Burning should be done in March or April before the wildfowl start nesting. He has reported this problem to Ducks Unlimited on several occasions over the last five years, and they are now watching the area. Last spring there was a lake fire that had, supposedly, been started accidentally by the exhaust of a tractor. Russell believes the fire was deliberately started. He finds it frustrating that those who get paid to protect the environment are not effective in preventing such occurrences. A few days after Russell told me this it was reported in the *Edmonton Journal* that Fish and Wildlife budgets had been cut and that fewer than one hundred officers are in the field to enforce wildlife regulations across Alberta.

The changes Russell has recommended point towards practical solutions to ecological problems. If we are to avoid the catastrophic ecological effects of economic activities that do not consider environmental assessment and planning, the public must pressure government and industry to respond to these issues. We can learn a great deal about wildlife management and nature conservation from people such as Russell who have firsthand experience of environmental problems and who are deeply concerned about the destruction of their homeland.

I will let Russell have the last word: 'What I can't understand is when they go logging in the Swan Hills or Hinton area, they leave the land next to broke; there are no trees there, no roots, herbs, nothing. Why don't they put the farmers there, since it's already cleared and wasted land anyway. They should put the farmers where the loggers have already done the damage. Then they try to plant little trees there. Why don't they just cut down and drag out the big trees they need without uprooting the entire area. If they left the smaller trees the wind wouldn't knock them down and the trees would regrow a lot faster. Even if the government says people and jobs come first, they still have to have respect for nature, because in the long run it works against people. They can't see the future. There's a lot of damage being done to the environment that should be discussed in order to realize what's happening to our country here. We call it the blessed country, but it sure is going to go back to rock in no time. I might not see that, but our great-grandchildren will.'

✹ Living with a
Medicine Man

Grant Ingram lived with the Williers in the summer of 1986, the year before Russell's father died. Grant was invited to stay in the Williers' guest bedroom. A reasonable payment was agreed upon for room and board and an informal contract negotiated. Grant assisted Russell in his work, as part payment both for room and board and for permission to do research. Grant's account of his experiences follows.

SANDRA

Soon after I arrived I had the opportunity to witness Russell's treatment of Sandra, a seven-year-old girl of East Indian background who had a severe case of psoriasis. Sandra's father, John, first heard about Russell in a Canadian Broadcasting Corporation news report and went to considerable lengths to find the healer.

Russell agreed to treat Sandra. Her family flew out from eastern Canada and borrowed a car from John's brother in Edmonton to make the four-hour drive to Sucker Creek. Since Sandra's family could stay only a short time, Russell planned to give Sandra an intensive treatment. She would be doctored every three hours around the clock. When her parents asked how long it would take for Sandra's psoriasis to go away, Russell reassured them that with the help of the Great Spirit it shouldn't take too long.

The first treatment took place later that day in the basement of Russell's house. Russell explained that this treatment would be the longest because Sandra must offer tobacco and a print to represent herself to the spiritual world. She selected a blue print. Fungus was lit and Sandra was instructed to undress and stand on the print. Praying in Cree, Russell walked around Sandra, purifying her psoriatic lesions with the smoke from the burning fungus. It was cold in the basement. Sandra shivered and appeared a little frightened. Her parents were present from the beginning, and they told her what Russell was about to do. Russell explained to Sandra that he would apply the herbal ointment starting from the top to the bottom of her body. He said that she must think about the Great Spirit: 'When you pray the smoke goes up into the sky, and the Great Spirit will help you. All kinds of wonders.' Russell talked in a gentle and reassuring voice. He explained to Sandra that he would do the first application of medicine but that afterwards her mother could do it. He told her that he would go into the forest to pray for her and offer the print and tobacco to the Great Spirit.

Sandra's parents were instructed to pray throughout the day. Sandra was told to drink as much medicated tea as possible in order to allow the tea to circulate throughout her body, particularly to the glands, the kidneys, the liver, and the bloodstream. This would allow the medicine to flush the psoriasis out of her system.

As the day progressed, John and his wife, Margerie, related the history of Sandra's psoriasis. It had started two years previously as a few tiny spots behind her ear. Sandra was taken to several skin specialists who were unable to help. Two weeks before their visit to Russell, Sandra came down with chicken-pox, and her psoriasis worsened and spread to most areas of her body.

The second application, three hours later, was supervised by Russell. Margerie applied the herbal solution. John said that they would stay for at least three days, and the solution would be applied every few hours in order to facilitate the healing process. John theorized about the healing process, using the analogy of a cancer. The cancer would be killed, allowing the surrounding cells to regenerate. Gradually, the afflicted areas would be reduced. The result would be that the skin would dry up and the scales would fall off as new skin appeared underneath. I asked John if he had gotten this idea from Russell. He said it was his own belief. It was remarkably similar to Russell's conception of the healing process.

After supper Russell and I drove over to see his parents and his brother Raymond. Raymond had ordered thirty-three head of cattle, which were being delivered by truck. There were extra cattle in the truck, so we had to unload the ones that didn't belong to Raymond first and hold them in an old corral while Raymond's cattle were unloaded. This took a long time. Russell was a little late getting back for Sandra's third herbal application. Russell explained to me that the spiritual introduction was accomplished, and the family could now apply the solution themselves, although he would be getting up early in the morning to make sure they did not miss the application. Russell mentioned that treating young children is much easier for him than treating adults. He becomes exhausted after treating elders, but dares not show it. If the patient perceives that the healer is not completely in control, he or she will become frightened, Russell explained.

Later that night, after Sandra's family had gone to bed, Russell discussed the forms of payment a native healer receives from patients. He referred to a native woman who had had cancer of the throat. Her throat had swollen to the point where she had difficulty swallowing, which is why she came for treatment. The woman died five months later, but she had been able to eat again and had actually gained weight because Russell had given her the right herb. The woman gave him fifty cents for payment, all she could afford. Russell emphasized that this was the way it should be. Adequacy of payment depends on circumstances. If, for example, someone goes to the bar or to play bingo on the weekend it is not right to give the medicine man only a few dollars. It is not right, either, if a person stays at Russell's house for four days, eats his food, and then gives him a mere twenty dollars. But there is nothing Russell can say, because a native healer cannot set a price.

Russell said that if he were to rely solely on his income as a medicine man he would not be able to support his family. He is forced to engage in a variety of activities in order to supplement his income from doctoring. He can't refuse patients who are broke. If he does this he is in trouble with the spiritual world. Russell said that if he could get a healing centre started on the reserve, he could be his own boss. He feels that this would be a lot better because he could put all his energy into healing and still be able to make a living.

Russell said that he was too busy these days. He was trying to raise money to buy a new trapline. He was involved with Moostoos Enterprises, a family corporation formed to construct an office building in a nearby town. He also wanted to complete a log house on a lot that the Williers own in Grouard. He told me that though these attempts to earn a decent living are frustrating at times they do make it possible for him to continue his healing activities. It is the miracles – the results of healing – that keep him going. He told me, 'I don't know which nationality would keep on like this, the way the native people have kept their culture in the face of adversity.'

Russell went downstairs to supervise the fourth application of the medicine. Sandra was shivering from the cold herbal solution, so Russell warmed it up on the stove before applying it. Later, when Sandra was asleep, her mother remarked that at about this time Sandra would usually be bleeding from scratching herself in her sleep. 'The itchiness has gone,' John said. 'She is not even moving in her sleep, so this is a nice sight.'

Later, while Russell, John, and I were talking, I mentioned the similarities between Russell's and John's beliefs in regard to healing. But there was one key difference. In John's experience, curers of East Indian descent in Tanzania will not accept direct payment for services. Instead, the patient is to pay the church. When I asked how the curers support themselves, he said they have ordinary jobs and businesses. When I asked if direct payment would spoil the power of a cure, he said that he didn't know for sure but he thought so, leaving me with the impression that he was uncertain about how to pay Russell for his services.

Russell cancelled the fifth application of herbs because Sandra was feeling feverish and was healing faster than he had expected anyway. There were pin-sized white spots of new skin forming in the infected areas.

John was able to resolve his dilemma over paying Russell. He was a natural handyman who often exchanged his services with others. He suggested to Russell that he could easily wire an old building on the property that Russell uses to store herbs and treat patients. John managed to wire the old building, hook up a doorbell and an outside floodlamp to the Willier residence, and improve the plumbing system. John's wife had helped with the cooking and cleaning and had prepared a special curry dinner one evening. They also bought a new toaster for Yvonne and gave Russell a small amount of money.

When Sandra's treatment was completed, she and her family left to visit relatives in Calgary, four hundred miles south of the Sucker Creek Reserve. Sandra, who had felt feverish while at the Willier's house, developed a high fever and was admitted to the hospital. Her parents did not tell the doctors of the recent treatment for psoriasis. Sandra received no medication, because the doctors did not know what was wrong with her. After a couple of days in the hospital her skin began to peel off in large strips, and she was left free of psoriasis. She returned to Toronto with her parents. After a time, some small lesions reappeared, so her father took her for a follow-up treatment at Sucker Creek. The lesions disappeared, and to the immense relief of the girl and her parents Sandra has been free of psoriasis for more than two years.

Russell takes care of the buffalo herd belonging to the Sucker Creek Band. One evening Russell and I went to check the fence surrounding the buffalo pound to make sure the herd was secure. Russell kept his eye out for deer and moose. He remarked that he would like to take his kids, Aron and Amy, to the nearby lake and just relax. I said that it sure gets hectic when he is doctoring someone. Russell agreed, saying that a medicine man is often called upon to drop everything and attend to a patient. He told me how much John had done around the place. I asked if this was satisfactory; or if he would have preferred more substantial payment. He said that it was fine, as John had done quite a lot of useful work.

Later that evening Russell, Yvonne, and I discussed the day's events around the kitchen table. Raymond's cattle, which were yearlings and quite wild, had broken out of the corral and scattered into the surrounding countryside. Russell, Raymond, Russell's other brother, Eddie, their father, and I had attempted unsuccessfully for four hours to round them up on horseback. We would gather some of them together, but at the first opportunity they would head for the bush. The cattle were capable of standing completely motionless while we rode past oblivious of their presence. All the while we were getting whacked in the head by branches and eaten alive by mosquitoes. I had ridden a horse only twice before in my life, and I could hardly walk later that day.

Russell sometimes complains about all the activities he must engage in to make a living, but he always seems to manage. This reflects an attitude towards work that I had never before encountered. Russell, who often works up to sixteen hours a day, does not appear to distinguish work from the rest of his life. On a given day Russell may be involved in four or five different projects and still manage to visit friends and relatives, play with his kids, go hunting, or do whatever else comes up. His schedule is flexible, and he does not pay much attention to the clock that governs non-native society. Russell works hard, and at this time we were working even harder than usual to finish up odds and ends so that Russell could commit himself more fully to spiritual matters.

SWEAT-LODGE

One day Russell decided to construct a new sweat-lodge and hold his first sweat of the season. Local helpers spent the day moving some rocks Russell had stockpiled to the new sweat-lodge site. While they were doing this Russell and I went to the buffalo pound area to collect willow saplings for construction of the lodge. Before cutting the saplings, Russell lit a piece of fungus, purified his hands, and prayed. He then purified his axe and offered tobacco to the spirit of the willow. We cut twenty straight willow saplings, leaving the branches on near the tips, and took them back to the sweat-lodge site half a mile behind the Willier house. Russell dug a hole about two and a half feet across and a foot and a half deep to hold the red-hot rocks used in the sweat-lodge ceremony. The hole was placed in the centre of the lodge site, and dirt was piled to the east of the site to form an altar. Russell planted the poles in a circle and bent the tips inward. Two saplings at a time were bent towards each other and joined, by twisting together the remaining branches, to form a hoop. When completed, the overlapping hoops created a dome approximately ten feet wide and five feet high. The dome was later covered with canvas.

Russell selected twenty-seven rocks, one for each willow pole used and seven for the most important Grandfathers, including Earth, Thunder, Lightning, Water, and Wind. He blessed five rocks, one for each of the cardinal directions and one for the sky. He placed all the rocks on a pile of logs east of the altar. More logs were stacked around the pyre and set on fire. Next came the preparation of the altar. Russell set a buffalo skull and some smaller bones on the dirt mound in front of the entrance to the sweat-lodge and placed several prints and a new stone pipe on top of the buffalo skull. The sweat-lodge, the altar, and the pile of burning logs were aligned to the east.

Russell then consecrated the sweat-lodge. Prints were purified and hung in each corner of the lodge: yellow prints in the east corner represented the Eagle Spirit, red prints in the south corner represented the Thunder Spirit, blue prints in the west corner represented the Bear Spirit, white prints in the north represented the Buffalo Spirit, and green prints in the centre represented Mother Earth. He also blessed several stone pipes and his medicine bundle with smoke from a burning fungus and placed them in the lodge, after which he circled the perimeter of the sweat-lodge inside and out in a clockwise direction with the fungus, praying. He then went on to arrange the inside of the altar. Old pipes were set on a light blue print, with an eagle wing on each side.

I was surprised when Russell placed a crucifix on top of the pipes. When I asked about the cross, Russell said he used it to represent the four directions. To one side of the blue print were four other prints, yellow, blue, green, and white. The new pipe was moved from the altar outside and placed on two coloured prints to the west of the first arrangement, and two pipes were placed on either side. All the pipes had been taken apart, with the stems placed beside the bowls, pointing east. The pipe on the right had a small leather medicine bag attached to it. At the base of the two old pipes were two unopened packages of tobacco. To the west of the tobacco were two rattles and a plastic bag containing herbs. During the sweat Russell was to break off pieces of these herbs and throw them on the hot rocks. Russell told me that someone had to be present at the sweat-lodge at all times once the fire was lit. He pointed out the various objects from his medicine bundle and asked me to note their position so he could see if anything had moved as a result of the ceremony.

The rocks were now hot and ready to be placed inside the hole in the centre of the lodge. This was my job. I brought one rock at a time on a pitchfork, walking from the pile of hot rocks past the buffalo skull on the right. After Russell had guided the rock into the hole I returned on the other side of the buffalo skull, moving in a clockwise direction, to get the next rock. On one trip when I forgot to 'walk with the sun' in this fashion, Russell warned me to 'back off' and I had to retrace my steps and start again. After the first five rocks were inside there was a break while Russell prayed. The remaining rocks were then brought inside.

We tried to get all the holes in the canvas covered so it would be completely dark inside. Then the first round began, a round dedicated to the elements. Wearing only shorts, we sat cross-legged on towels. I was stationed beside the door so I could open and close the flaps. Russell was on the other side closer to the rocks. He sang and prayed while dipping a cup into the bucket of water beside him. He threw the water over the white-hot rocks. The resulting blast of steam was so hot I nearly panicked. It took an effort of will to remain inside. As soon as the round was complete (I cannot remember much of this round as I was concentrating all my energy on not panicking), we both crawled out of the entrance and collapsed on the ground. Russell said that a new sweat is always harder on a person because many rocks are needed to bless the elements and willow saplings. He said that the spirits had almost entered during that round. While we were recuperating he told me that when the spirits arrive it feels as if your stomach suddenly leaves you.

The second round was dedicated to the willows and to the rocks themselves. Russell said this was to be a hot one, as there were many rocks and willows. I could not imagine anything hotter than the previous round. Russell prayed and sang for a time and then had a sudden coughing spell, which left him unable to continue singing. When the round was over we again collapsed outside on the ground. Russell was upset that he hadn't been able to finish his singing during that round.

I asked what the next round was to be for. He replied, 'It's for us.' Russell prayed and sang again while dousing the rocks periodically with water. He announced in a loud voice, 'Thunder Spirit we request your presence!' Wings could be heard flapping. The rattles began to sound, accompanied by flashes of phosphorescent light. Russell had instructed me beforehand to think of the Great Spirit and concentrate on any personal problems I was facing. He had told me that I shouldn't be concerned if he stopped singing, as he sometimes goes into a trance when the spirits come. Russell stopped singing and began to hyperventilate. He then told me, in a strange voice, that I was having a hard time believing. He said that he was going to ask the spirit whether or not I was learning anything.

The Thunder Spirit replied that I was thinking about my girlfriend too much and that I was preoccupied with alcohol. If I wanted to learn, the spirit said, I needed to 'smarten up'!

Russell said that the spirit wouldn't stay long because the tarp was too full of holes. He was asked by the spirit to sing. He sang, and the round was over. This round had been very impressive for me. I was in a mood to suspend my normal beliefs, and I remembered that I had indeed been thinking of my drinking problem and my relationship with my girl-friend. I told Russell I really did want to learn and that I didn't want my drinking problem to interfere. I felt close to Russell at this moment. I remember thinking that the trauma of undergoing a sweat breaks down normal barriers of defensiveness. I was very pleased to have made it through three rounds.

In the fourth and final round, Russell began praying and singing. A loud clicking noise occurred and lasted for several seconds. Russell fanned the rocks with the eagle wings. The resulting blast of heat felt good. When the final round was over, I opened the entrance and we both went outside to recuperate.

We rested briefly. Russell asked me to go inside and collect the four prints he had hung from willow branches in each of the four corners at the top of the lodge. This had to be done in sequence, again going clockwise. I brought out the new pipe and a package of tobacco. We smoked the pipe sitting on an old car seat that had been placed nearby. Russell took a long time, offering the pipe in the different directions and praying. When I asked what the words to his prayer were, he said that it was like asking the spirits to take up a message to God. I was offered the pipe three times and told to concentrate again on what I had been thinking about before the spirit entered. He told me that the smoke coming from a person's mouth is believed to rise up as a prayer to the Great Spirit.

Later that evening while we were having supper, Russell said that he would ask the Beaver Spirit to come to his next sweat so we would be able to complete everything we had planned for the summer. He told Yvonne that in a few weeks they would be receiving word that Moostoos Enterprises had received a government grant. When Yvonne asked how he knew this, Russell smiled and pointed up.

Before becoming acquainted with Russell Willier I believed myself to be an atheist. I thought that the 'anthropological imagination' would allow me to empathize with any belief different from my own. My position has since shifted from atheism to agnosticism, a transition that is, for me at least, quite radical. Russell seems to be tolerant towards non-natives who are seeking exposure to native religion. In a sweat-lodge ceremony I attended, Russell relayed a message from the spirits to the effect that I wanted to believe and that because of my upbringing in another culture my scepticism was to be expected. Russell's philosophy implies that until a person is ready nothing is going to happen, so why try and force someone to change?

The following incidents occurred in connection with various sweat-lodge ceremonies.

Russell planned to hold a sweat for some people who were coming from Edmonton. We were about to begin preparations when Russell received a long-distance phone call. It was from one of the men in Edmonton who had requested the sweat. They had not left yet and did not think that they had enough money to make the trip. Russell said that they should come anyway and that he would pay for their gas home.

It was getting late, and Russell knew that he had to begin the ceremony before dark or evil spirits could enter the lodge. Judging from the position of the sun I felt there was no chance that the guests from Edmonton would arrive in time. We waited for as long as we could and then began the ceremony. We had a young boy as doorman. As payment for his services, Russell gave him free movies and the use of a video machine.

We had completed one round and were well into the second when the sound of flapping wings was heard near the entrance to the lodge. Russell had earlier placed medicine pipes on top of his eagle wings and had fashioned a sweeper from willow stems and leaves to clean the debris from the hot rocks that were brought in. As a sceptic, I naturally assumed that this is what was used to create the sound of flapping wings. But Russell said the Eagle Spirit had told him that it was waiting for the people to arrive and that they 'were right around the corner.' When the round was over Russell and I went to the doorway to get some air, and within five minutes the people from Edmonton arrived. Russell and I looked at each other and laughed.

On another occasion Russell declared that he was going to have a family sweat. I wasn't sure what he meant by this, or if I would be able to participate, so I just waited to see what would develop. We started to get the wood ready. Russell told me to pretend he was my helper. This, he believed, would be the best way for me to learn. Since I didn't know the entire procedure, I waited for cues from Russell. I was learning, though, and when we finished Russell said, 'You're starting to master it, little by little, even the door.' I had been having difficulties covering the entrance in order to block the light.

Russell prepared his medicine bundle. He seemed to do a lot more praying and purification that day. Always passing the burning fungus in a clockwise direction, he paid careful attention to each item in his bundle in the sweat-lodge. We went outside and waited for the rocks to turn white-hot. Russell told me to go to the house and tell Yvonne to phone the people who were coming to the sweat. Yvonne, who had just woken from a nap, said she didn't know whom to phone and that if they were coming to the sweat then they would come. I asked who was supposed to be coming, and she said, 'His sisters or something.' I told Russell what had happened and he just said, 'Oh.'

I passed all the rocks inside to Russell, and we went outside to wait for a while. It seemed that no one was coming to the sweat. I was sprawled beside an old car seat. Russell sat on a tree trunk. After we had been quiet for quite a long time, Russell asked me what I would do if the prime minister or another important person were coming to the sweat. I thought about it, then said that I didn't place one person above another. I mumbled that the prime minister is a person like anyone else. Russell rephrased the question to get his point across: if someone was coming whom I really respected, would I try to do as good a job as I could or would I just lie there sprawled out on the ground?

Russell talked about how best to encourage the spirits to be present. He asked me if a spirit in search of a warrior would choose someone who was just lying around. He answered his own question: 'No! Because such a warrior wouldn't last. He would be killed. The spirit would choose the one who is alert, the one who is strong.'

He talked about how important it is to conduct oneself properly and how the right attitude has to be developed over an entire lifetime. Russell described some of the sweats he had been to where everyone was joking around all the time. He asked what I thought would happen and went on to say that the spirits wouldn't come. 'It's as simple as that,' he stated. He made it clear that if he went to someone's house and they didn't show him any respect he wouldn't go back. 'It's the same with the spirits,' he said. 'They don't have to come.'

Russell will not return to someone's sweat if he sees disrespectful behaviour, though he said it is perfectly all right to have a joke or laugh if it comes up naturally; the spirits understand. I told Russell that I had understood his message. He said, 'You're slowly being introduced, you're getting the puzzle together bit by bit.'

We began the sweat. The first two rounds were uneventful. In the third round the spirits told him to look to the clouds for a sign. When we went outside, I was standing by myself, looking around. I remember being impressed with how pure everything looked. Russell was lying down outside near the entrance to the sweat-lodge. He told me to come over, saying that the spirits had given him a sign. He then pointed up at the clouds and said, 'See the pipe?'

I was amazed to see a pipe-shaped cloud passing above us, with a puff of smoke coming out of the bowl. Russell interpreted this sign to mean that we were to smoke the pipe then, not after the last round, as is customary. He explained that the pipe ceremony would be for his sisters, who had not been able to come to the ceremony.

MY RELATIONSHIP WITH RUSSELL

I regret that I wasn't able to be more open-minded in regard to what Russell was attempting to impart to me. There is no way now to determine what doors might have been opened to me had my attitudes been more compatible with native spiritual beliefs.

Personality differences between myself and Russell became apparent as field-work progressed. It is safe to say that we do things in very different ways. Russell prefers to jump right in and get tasks accomplished, whereas I prefer to think things out beforehand. It might be said that our coping styles differ, and that I am far more introverted.

Looking back, I think a large part of the problem may have been due to my wanting to play the role of anthropologist. And I would at times be angry at Russell for his lack of sensitivity about what I was really like. I felt at times that I couldn't be myself in his presence. I often resented the role I had taken on, experiencing displeasure over the phoney way I perceived myself to be acting at times. When really in a state of funk I would blame my unhappiness on Russell, feeling I wasn't getting any new 'material.' When I thought I couldn't stand it any longer, Russell would tell me something that would open a new dimension of understanding. It was uncanny. It is likely that Russell was constantly testing me. He had predicted that there would be times when I would think I was not learning anything new, though I really was.

Personal differences have a way of becoming exaggerated when one is doing field-work, and there reached a point where I believed my presence to be the cause of conflict. This came to a head one night after a sweat-lodge ceremony with many different visitors. David Young and his son, Chris, had just left for Edmonton after a week's visit, and Russell was getting ready to set out on a trip to the next province to doctor a new patient. I was to accompany him. The time was one o'clock in the morning. Everyone had gone to bed, and Russell and I were sitting at the kitchen table having tea. I felt that the time was right to present Russell with a pouch of tobacco I had been saving for him. I believed, at this time, that I had seriously jeopardized my relationship with the Williers by my mood swings and periodic drinking. I was relieved when Russell, after receiving the tobacco – and listening to an account of my self-doubts – informed me that he had been aware of our differences in personality and behaviour all along and that I was not to worry. He said that I had helped out more than I could know.

Being a guest in the family home and at the same time recording all my observations turned out to be a problem. I had been advised to keep a private field-work journal where matters of a more personal nature could be recorded. But my field notes soon came to consist of both professional and personal observations. I had broken the rule of keeping confidential material separate from my field notes. That Russell and Yvonne would want to read my field notes had not occurred to me. But that is exactly what they requested.

When I complied with their request and they started reading through my notes, they were shocked to discover that I had recorded things that were really none of my business. I had thought I was doing a good job by recording everything; instead I had become, particularly in Yvonne's eyes, a 'spy' within the family. The responsibility that comes with being allowed into other people's lives is something that cannot be grasped by reading a textbook.

Problems like the one I caused are seldom written about in the anthropological literature. This is changing, as the people with whom anthropologists have traditionally worked demand to be full partners in the research process and to have their points of view voiced. Anthropologists and other social scientists must take responsibility for their actions, not as so-called impartial observers, but as human beings who have a direct impact on the people with whom they work, and who in turn are changed as a result of their experiences. We will return to this theme in the last chapter.

❧ Native
Medicine for
Non-Natives

Russell encouraged us, in 1984, to document his treatment of skin diseases. This was a rare opportunity for us, since Indian medical procedures have rarely been documented and most medicine men are reluctant to discuss practices that have a history of being mocked and ridiculed by non-native people. Russell feels strongly that Indian medicine and Indian religion are powerful and that it is his duty to demonstrate as much. Russell, moreover, is very concerned about young natives who show little interest or pride in native ways, specifically in native medicine. He believes that if scientific investigation can 'prove' the effectiveness of native medicine it might help change the attitudes of native young people and encourage them to return to the Sweetgrass Trail. It is his hope that a return to the Sweetgrass Trail will reduce the alcoholism and suicide rampant on many reserves.

Russell's decision to allow his medical practices to be documented has been controversial in the native community. He defends his decision in the following way: 'There are a lot of problems facing natives today, which is why I am willing to bring Indian medicine out in the open. Our culture is slowly dying. Even our language is dying. We're losing a lot of young people who could be on the Sweetgrass Trail. Many are not proud of being Indian and so they get into alcohol, they get into drugs, and some commit suicide or get run over in vehicle accidents. So if we can bring back pride to the young ones, as they grow up they will have a better chance to make a good living. The elders are trying to help, but they're not open enough.

'Another reason is that native medicine has been used for years and years, centuries, to help people and to cure diseases, but because it has never been recorded, we're losing a lot of the knowledge and fewer people are practising it. In our reserve there's hardly anyone who knows anything about it. The young generation don't know too much about it, and the elders are slowly dying off. Sometimes a fifty-year-old man may go back to it, but it's already too late for him to master everything in his lifetime. There are some very powerful medicine men practising today, but they're not interested in teaching. The natives who have this power and knowledge should try to put up a school and try to teach those of the younger generation who are interested. I have heard the elders say that although it's underground now, one day it will be out in the open, and when that day comes there will be a lot of people seeking it and many will be healed. Some of these elders told me that they would be more open about if if they knew enough English, but that right now they aren't ready to become involved since they wouldn't be able to answer questions if they didn't understand exactly what was being asked.

'There are some natives who are very worried that the herbal combinations are being recorded and passed over to the white society, but that's not the case. We're simply trying to prove that we've got a religion and that it's powerful. We're not passing our medicines over to anybody except the native youth who want to learn. You can't just pass it over to anyone you wish, anyway. The person has to be chosen by the spiritual world. Natives should be aware that if we don't do this, the culture itself is slowly going to die out. We should pull together, instead of disagreeing with each other's ideas, and try to help ourselves and others. If we don't work together, we're not going to accomplish anything.

'Another thing is that native medicine can cure many diseases, as can Western doctors. They should work together, have a system so that, when non-native doctors know that native medicine can cure some diseases that they don't handle well, they should refer the patient to a native medicine man. For example, sometimes when a person has sugar diabetes and he's starting to break out around the ankles, the doctor recommends cutting his leg off to prevent the spread of gangrene. But sugar diabetes sores are not that hard to cure. I have doctored patients who would probably have lost their legs, but when we started using herbal medicine, the diabetes sores got better. I can't cure diabetes, but I can heal the sores and keep it at a level where the blood pressure doesn't go up. If non-native doctors knew that we can cure sugar diabetes sores, they would have to think before they recommended amputation.

'Most natives don't hesitate to refer their patients to Western doctors. When someone comes to us, say with a broken bone, we send him to the hospital where he can be x-rayed. The doctors can put the bone back together way better than we can. The same is true of penicillin. If someone has real bad bronchitis or pneumonia, we send him to the western doctor so he can start getting his shots. We're trying to make sure a person gets the best care. I would like Western doctors to accept what we are and what we can do instead of having conflict with us. We should pull together.

'A lot of people don't know how powerful native medicine can be and the diseases we can cure. Partly this is because of phoney medicine men who are in it for the money. For example, if someone with a lot of faith in Indian medicine went to one of these phonies who doesn't know how to heal, how will he feel when there are no results and he's paid a lot of money? Do you think he'll go to another medicine man? These phoney medicine men are the ones who are ruining it, because they're not sincere and most of them are there to make a fast dollar. Some of them use magician's tricks, and that's not right because the real medicine men don't need that in order to heal. When a person gets doctored, you'll see the results, you don't need anything else. If a person gets better, he usually tells another person that this particular medicine man cured him. That's how it went around the country for the last few hundred years. That's where the good healers get their advertisement. Maybe when it's out in the open, this will prevent the phonies from practising and thereby giving Indian medicine a bad reputation.'

Before becoming involved in the Psoriasis Research Project, Russell consulted the elders on his reserve as well as his spirit helpers. He asked for guidance and confirmation that it was appropriate for him to demonstrate the power of his medicine. Some elders were against the project, while others supported it. Most important for Russell, however, was the positive answer he received from the spirit world. He decided to proceed.

Russell claims to have cures for a variety of diseases. We chose to document his treatment of psoriasis, since visible lesions could be monitored effectively throughout the treatment period. Psoriasis is a chronic skin disease the cause of which is not well understood. The symptoms vary from small isolated patches of red skin to thick, scaly lesions covering most of the body. From 2 to 6 per cent of North Americans suffer from psoriasis. There is no known cure, and the best that Western doctors can do is to treat the lesions. Although psoriasis is not life-threatening, it can be very unsightly and extremely itchy. The psychological consequences can be overwhelming. One patient, for example, reported that, when he took the bus, nearby passengers would move away from him, and he would sometimes be asked if he had leprosy. Another patient reported that whenever she went to the local swimming-pool with her children during the summer other swimmers immediately left the water. Sufferers try various therapies, orthodox and unorthodox. Unfortunately, many of the present methods of treatment have unpleasant and sometimes serious side-effects.

PILOT STUDY

The research team was headed by David Young and included Janice Morse from the Faculty of Nursing at the University of Alberta, Ruth McConnell from the Provincial Museum of Alberta, and Lise Swartz, the author of this chapter. We were assisted by medical doctors, chemists, and a professional video crew. Our documentation encompassed initial assessment of potential patients, treatment sessions in an inner-city health clinic, sweat-lodge ceremonies on a site near Edmonton, a thanking ceremony, and final evaluation. Research began with a pilot study, involving two patients who were treated between November and December 1984. Both patients showed improvement, and we decided to continue the research with a larger group of patients. From March to June 1985 eleven patients were treated for psoriasis.

To prove or disprove the efficacy of native medicine in alleviating or curing psoriasis it is necessary to use control groups, so that treated and untreated patients can be compared. Because of the large number of people required to set up a valid research design, however, the use of elaborate controls was not feasible for our research. Moreover, Russell made it clear that he wanted no part of an experiment in which people were treated like 'guinea pigs.' But Russell did allow us to control the research environment to a certain extent and to record the results in detail. He allowed the research to be conducted in a clinic with medical doctors present as observers, and he allowed us to photograph and videotape patients' progress.

Five patients volunteered to participate in the pilot study, which began in November 1984 at the Boyle McCauley Health Centre in Edmonton. Obtaining permission to conduct the research required some time, as the staff were uncertain about the appropriateness of having this kind of research done at their clinic. They eventually called the College of Physicians and Surgeons to ask permission, and it was granted, much to everyone's surprise. The clinic had a large meeting room in which the entire group could assemble for discussion, ceremonies, and treatment, a smaller room across the hall that could be used for photography, and a space where patients could be interviewed privately.

On the first day of the experiment the research team and the patients arrived at the clinic at around three o'clock in the afternoon. The agenda for this session included examination of the patients by the physicians, photographing of the patients' skin lesions, and an explanation by Russell of his healing procedures. Russell encouraged both the patients and members of the research team to ask questions. Initially, I was apprehensive about interviewing Russell. What kinds of questions were relevant? What were the sensitive issues? Would a medicine man be willing to answer questions posed by a woman? My anxieties were put to rest as I talked to Russell. We soon established a rapport, and I discovered I could ask anything that came to mind. If he didn't want to answer he would laugh, joke, or state simply, 'I can't tell you that.'

We were all seated in a large circle, and Russell began to explain his medicine to us: 'For the Great Spirit, the problems you have are nothing. He can cure them easily. But I need your mind, and your faith, and your confidence. Everything will come through the power of the Great Spirit. He might test your faith. He might make your disease worse for a few days just to test you out. You might get scared if you think it's going to get worse, but you have to have faith in yourself, in God, and in the power of the herbs. He has planted these herbs all over the world for people to use. They're not mine or any medicine man's. They're taken from Mother Earth and combined into medicines to help cure your sickness.'

Russell went on to say that when someone comes to him for treatment she or he must present him with a package of cigarette tobacco and a cotton print in one of the yellow, red, blue, white, and green colours of the earth. The tobacco is given to Mother Earth whenever herbs are taken, and the cloth is hung in the bush as an offering to the spirit helpers. These offerings open the doors to the spirit world and provide a pathway for healing powers to flow through the medicine man to patients. Russell said that without these offerings he would not have the power to heal. Even if he recognized that someone in his own family suffered from a sickness and needed treatment that he knew he could provide, he could not volunteer to help unless the person made the request by giving Russell tobacco and a print. He emphasized that payment for cures must be a genuine expression of gratitude. 'It was never told to us by the Great Spirit to set a price,' he said. 'It was up to the person and must come from the heart. What I always say is if a person can't give anything, at least buy a coffee just to show appreciation.'

Yvonne Willier said, 'At one time you offered a cherished four-legged animal, such as a horse, cow, or hunting dog. But it's not that way anymore because lots of people don't have access to these animals. If you have something in your house that you want to give, or money, it's up to you.'

Laughing, Russell pointed out that 'the vehicle represents the four-legged animal nowadays.'

Russell told the patients: 'Now you may have some doubts during the next six weeks, or you may want to back out. You can quit any time. It's your decision. Some of you will probably get results right away while others won't because of lack of faith. But if you see your neighbour here and he's getting fast results, that's to help you to have a little more faith in the medicine. Often it's better to treat several people together where they can see one another. So I hope it will benefit all of us who are here today. I want to start with smoking the fungus here, and to say a prayer. You'll pray in your own way, but we'll have to walk this incense around the room first.'

Yvonne, with a smouldering piece of fungus on a plate, went around to each participant. 'What I'm burning here,' she said, 'is called a fungus. We use it for incense. It purifies the air, it purifies your body, and also, as the smoke rises into heaven, your prayers and wishes will be carried with the smoke. So what you should do now, if everybody wants to participate, is to catch the smoke and spread it on yourselves. That will purify your body so the herbs can penetrate.'

'As you know,' Russell took up the explanation, 'when you want the spirits to come, you purify the place like we just did and then you'll ask the spirits to tell God how grateful we are. Now I'm going to pray my way, and you pray your way. It's still the same God.'

When Russell finished praying in Cree, the patients went upstairs to be diagnosed and assessed by two doctors who worked at the clinic. The patients then returned to Russell for diagnosis and evaluation of their condition. Only two of the five patients were told to return for treatment: Karen, a young mother with a six-year history of psoriasis on her knees and elbows, and Bob, a middle-aged man with a fifteen-year history of severe psoriasis on his elbows, knees, ears, and scalp. Russell suggested that two patients could come for treatment in the spring should their condition worsen. 'I usually don't take them when they're mild cases,' Russell explained. 'I send them to the doctor. If it was real serious I would doctor them, but for these mild ones I would recommend they keep seeing whoever they're seeing now and be thankful to the spirits that it's not serious. And the other patient whose psoriasis is pretty severe has just started on a new medication. He'll always think that it is actually his new medication that's curing him, so I won't try to doctor him, as he wouldn't have much confidence in the herbs. If he tries his new medication for maybe another two or three years and his psoriasis won't go away, he can come back. As far as Bob is concerned, he's had it since 1958 so he knows it won't leave the system. He'll have faith in the herbs.'

'How fast, on average,' one of us asked, 'would patients start to see some results?'

'When they're really bad you can see results very soon, in about a week,' Russell replied. 'With these cases it might be slower because they're very light and the lesions are not flared up. When it's flared, it's easier to cure.'

'I think,' interjected Yvonne, 'it's the case that a lot of people don't turn to Indian medicine until they're desperate. They've tried everything, and it won't go away. Then they turn to Indian medicine. That's why Russell usually gets the bad cases.'

'Do you see some of those same skin diseases up north that are a lot worse?' asked one of the doctors who had come down to take part in the discussion.

'Yes,' answered Russell, 'they're a lot worse. But usually when we doctor them they don't get it back like they do down here. We've treated many people up north who didn't have to return to their regular doctor. Once they start the herbal medication, they improve and it doesn't come back.'

The other doctor stated, 'It will come back. It is very rarely cured.'

'I've had people who looked like they were painted with red paint come for treatment and they're one hundred per cent now,' Russell replied. 'A few spots appeared maybe a year after I treated them, and I gave them a little more herbal medication and it has never returned. That was four or five years ago. But I know a lot of the native patients are sent here to see the skin specialist and they are told that it is in the native blood, which is why they can't get rid of it. That's what the majority told me. They would spend two to three years on medication, but they would never improve. The medicine that they would get would do a lot of good at the time, but the psoriasis would always come back when they stopped using the medicine. Couldn't seem to get rid of it completely. But you will see, it can be cured.'

Russell explained that psoriasis has a contagious element, meaning that it is both hidden in the bloodstream and visible on the surface of the skin. For this reason, treating the symptoms alone will not cure psoriasis. Treatment must be directed towards purifying the blood. The herbal tea purifies the blood and at the same time forces the poison or infectious agent to the surface of the skin. A herbal solution that is intended to kill germs is then applied to the lesions. Russell informed the two patients that they should return the next day with their tobacco and print offerings. He would then doctor them by having them drink a herbal tea and rubbing a herbal solution on their lesions.

The first treatment session was held at the clinic the following day, 23 November 1984. The room was purified by passing incense around three times in a clockwise direction. Russell purified himself by chewing a bitter herb, which he then rubbed over his face, arms, and hands. After this he drew the fungus smoke toward his upper body with his cupped hands, an action he later explained as 'lending your hands out to the spiritual world.' Purification acts as a shield – almost like invisible gloves – to protect the healer from disease. Although it was hardly noticeable, and then only to someone who was watching his face very closely, Russell entered an altered state of consciousness during this ritual. Discussing the intensity that is required of him during doctoring, Russell said that after a ceremony he must 'paddle back to himself' to regain equilibrium. Russell jokes a lot after a ceremony, which is probably one way of paddling back.

Bob was the first patient to arrive. He had the tobacco offering, but no print. Russell did not find this surprising. He had, in fact, anticipated it and brought a blue print along. Russell said, 'If I told Bob that the Great Spirit will cure him within a week or more he'd probably laugh in my face, because he's had psoriasis for fifteen years. I have to work slowly to open his eyes to what's going to take place and to accept it, and that's very hard, especially since he has doubts about it. For example, if these two people came to my home I wouldn't doctor them the same night. I would wait until the next day. I would first have to make them feel at home, try to open their minds to the situation, make them feel comfortable. You have to bring them to the point where they have faith in you and the powers of the Great Spirit, and that takes time.'

Bob was asked to stand on his print. Russell told him the meaning of the ritual and its symbols. He said, 'What you're doing is representing yourself to the spirit world when you stand on the cloth.' Russell sprinkled the tobacco in a circle around Bob's feet and prayed in Cree. Both the print and tobacco had been purified by passing them over burning incense. Bob was asked to step off the print and sit down while Russell proceeded to apply the herbal solution to the lesions. While doing this, he talked to Bob, describing how the treatment works, citing past examples of cures, and reassuring him that he too would be cured if he would drink the tea regularly and apply the solution. Bob must have come to trust Russell somewhat during this short period because he started telling him many episodes from his own life, a life filled with hardships and difficulties. When Russell had finished applying the herbal solution to all the lesions, Bob reported feeling numb and tingling.

When Bob was finished, the print, with the tobacco inside, was tied into a bundle. It was to be hung in the bush, on Russell's property, until some natural event such as a fire or decay would eventually destroy it. 'The faster you hang the prints, the better the healing,' Russell said. Herbal tea, which had been boiling in an adjacent room, was then offered, not only to Bob but also to the four researchers. Russell's words were reassuring: 'It's got a reasonable flavour to it. You'll drink it with your tea. Throw two of these herbs in your tea pot, let it boil real good and then add your tea. It will look lumpy and sticky like tongue that's cooked and you can actually apply that right onto the sores after it has boiled. This tea will help purify your blood but it can also be used to apply right on the lesion to absorb and suck out some of the poison.'

Karen, who presented Russell with a white print, was treated in much the same way as Bob. Appointment times were made for follow-up documentation of the patients' lesions. It was arranged that Russell would return in two weeks for the second treatment session.

A few days later Bob and Karen came to the university so that we could document any changes that had occurred in their lesions. 'Russell said it would flare up,' commented Bob, 'and it did yesterday, but it's a lot better than it was. I used to wake up at night and itch, and now I don't itch at all. I came home, put the stuff on, and no itch. Before I would come home and scratch. And at night it would scale and fall off in the morning, but this morning it didn't peel off. Before it would be very thick and you could just rip it right off. Even my ears, which were all covered, are better. The stuff stinks like heck, but who cares as long as it gets rid of the psoriasis.'

Karen agreed: 'I also find that the itchiness has decreased, but sometimes it burns when I apply the solution. It's really hard to put it on all the time because I have two night classes. The smell is so bad that one day I washed with tomato juice to try to get rid of it.'

The second treatment session occurred twelve days later, again in the Boyle McCauley Health Centre. Russell first examined the patients and noted their improvement. The physician agreed that some improvement had occurred: 'It certainly is less aggressive.

The reduction in size is not dramatic, but certainly the redness and the scaling are less.'

Patients were requested to keep drinking the herbal tea but to discontinue use of the herbal solution unless new lesions appeared or existing lesions flared up. Patients were informed that they could add a teaspoon of vinegar to 'cut down the smell' of the solution. They were given goose grease to make the skin more supple. Russell emphasized the importance of allowing the body to take over and 'heal on its own.'

Before completing the second treatment session, Russell prayed to thank the Great Spirit for the improvement in the patients' conditions. He first lit a piece of fungus and purified his hands over it, then passed smouldering sage around the room three times, clockwise. Russell then purified the goose grease over incense and pointed it in the four cardinal directions. He chanted a prayer in Cree, accompanying this with the steady shaking of his rattle. The session was concluded. He promised to return in two weeks, at which time he felt the patients would be healed and 'probably would have nothing to come for.'

When Russell returned for the final session, which included a ceremony to give thanks to the Great Spirit for curing the patients, only Karen showed up. Russell's disappointment was evident, particularly since Bob had reported to Russell on the previous day that his psoriasis was much better. Bob left without giving Russell a forwarding address. It may have been that Bob was simply not able to offer any gift to Russell. This is unfortunate, since Russell would have accepted a cup of coffee, for example, as a token of gratitude.

Karen certainly had improved, but it could not be claimed that she had been cured. Russell said the slowness in her recovery was possibly due to the fact that her lesions were not active at the time of treatment: 'They were on low profile, and they're easier to get rid of when they're flared up.' One of the researchers reminded Russell that neither patient had participated in a sweat-lodge ceremony as originally had been suggested. He agreed that 'it could make the difference,' because 'in the sweat-lodge your skin pores open up,' allowing the solution to seep into the infected skin areas to kill the infectious agent. Although improvement in Karen's condition was not as good as Russell had anticipated, we found the therapeutic outcome encouraging.

FURTHER RESEARCH

In March 1985 fifteen patients were recruited through advertisements in local newspapers. Although Russell knew that he might not have enough herbs for so many people, he felt it impossible to turn anyone away. However, after explaining the principles of his treatment method to the patients, he indicated that, initially, he would treat only the three patients who were most severely afflicted with psoriasis. The patients were chosen, and we arranged to conduct the first treatment the following day.

Unfortunately, Russell and Yvonne received a telephone call from the reserve the next day requesting them to return home immediately, since Yvonne's brother had been killed in a snowmobile accident. This was to be followed by other misfortunes, eventually leading Russell and Yvonne to question the wisdom of continuing the experiments. The first treatment session was cancelled, and Russell abandoned his plans to treat only the most severe patients. The eleven patients who still wished to take part in the experiment were rescheduled for two weeks later.

When Russell returned to Edmonton, Yvonne, who was to have been his assistant, was unable to attend because she could not break the taboo prohibiting menstruating women from being present at a healing ceremony.

The session began with purification of the room. Russell purified himself and told me, his assistant, how to purify my hands. This was done by chewing a bitter herb, which was then rubbed over my hands and up my arms to the elbows where Russell had drawn a circle around my arm with red ochre. The herb was terribly bitter and caused me some discomfort and nausea. I had visions of vomiting, with the video capturing every detail, and I was worried about ruining the religious nature of the ritual. Russell was aware of my predicament, saying that it would soon pass. He then purified the pipe over the smoking incense, praying intently in Cree. It was difficult, when Russell was deeply concentrating on the spiritual world and its sacred symbols, to decide whether it was appropriate to take photographs. Clicks and flashing lights seemed incompatible with the religious atmosphere. Since our intention was to document everything, however, pictures were taken. Once the preparations were completed and all participants were seated, the pipe was passed around the circle of participants three times, with the comment from Russell that 'if it runs out of tobacco, it'll still have to go around.'

The male patients were treated by Russell, and the female patients were treated by me according to Russell's instructions. The male patients presented their prints and tobacco offerings. These were purified over incense and placed on the floor, their placement determined by their colour. The tobacco was placed on the prints, and patients were requested to stand on their prints, facing in one of the four directions. While they all remained standing, Russell doctored each patient individually. Incense was placed at the patients' feet to purify the tobacco and herbal solution. Tobacco was sprinkled around the patients' feet in a clockwise direction while Russell prayed in Cree. We then proceeded to apply the herbal solution to lesions on the patients, starting from the top of the body and moving down, circling each patient to daub the lesions three times. All eleven patients received treatment in this manner.

The room was thick with incense. Russell joked with the patients, who were joking among themselves. The group was eventually to become very close – perhaps it was a relief to communicate and share the sufferings that they had experienced as a result of psoriasis. They developed a liking for Russell and a respect for what he was doing. Often they would comment on how much they had improved, despite the lack of visible changes in their lesions. Once, when one of the physicians came down to see how things were progressing, he mentioned that he felt like an intruder in our tight-knit group. It was rare for a patient to fail to show up for a session.

The second treatment session, which occurred a week later,

was more informal. Following purification of the hands, Russell treated the male patients while I applied the herbal solution to the females. This time males and females were treated together in the same room. Women requiring privacy were taken behind a screen.

The third treatment session was different. The meeting room was again used, and this time was divided by a large screen. Russell treated the male patients on one side of the screen, while Yvonne treated the female patients on the other side. In addition to the usual treatment, the eagle ceremony was performed on two male patients, one of whom had expressed scepticism regarding the effectiveness of the treatment. The other patient's psoriasis was the most severe, with lesions spread all over his body.

The eagle ceremony was performed in the following way. Two eagle wings, which had been wrapped in yellow cloth, were purified by passing them above smouldering incense, as Russell prayed in Cree. Holding one wing in each hand, he proceeded to flutter these about the patient's body. He started at the front and walked in a circle around the patient, briefly touching the patient's body with the tips of the wings. Kneeling, Russell prayed once more as he passed the wings above the incense and again wrapped them in their yellow cloth.

Following the ceremony, one of the patients told us what he felt: 'It was a good feeling. I didn't find it odd at all; you can understand what's happening. It's never a question, you know, but that the thing makes sense, given its own framework. The wings do make a difference on the person they're being used on. There's absolutely no question that that odd touch they have is quite distinctive, and it feels as if you're about to take off and there's also the sound they make. A little touch here and there, but not every time, and you can hear this, whatever, flying near you and just touching you every once in a while, so that the mental picture is very strong.'

One patient who reported that his condition had worsened began to have serious doubts about the treatment, which he communicated to the others. His negative attitude was resented, and Russell tried hard to explain to him that in the initial stages of treatment the lesions often become more inflamed and that he should consider this as a positive sign that the herbs were working to push the disease from the blood to the skin. The patient, however, decided not to continue treatment, bringing the numbers in the group to ten.

The next stage involved a sweat-lodge ceremony. On 20 April all the patients and researchers met at the Provincial Museum in Edmonton at six o'clock in the morning to drive to the Sucker Creek Reserve for the sweat. No one had expected a major snow-storm at this time of year, but that is what we got. The roads were almost impassable, so we decided to postpone the trip. One of us joked that perhaps the spirits were not prepared to receive so many visitors at this particular time.

Because of the difficult logistics involved in moving the project north, Russell decided to construct a sweat-lodge on David Young's property, a forty-minute drive from Edmonton. One week after the cancelled trip to the reserve, Russell arrived at David's place, having gotten up at dawn to meditate for several hours. He brought along a nephew to help him build the lodge.

It took Russell, his nephew, and David most of the day to prepare for the sweat, as willows had to be cut, rocks collected, and the herbs prepared. Patients arrived around three o'clock in the afternoon. They had been instructed to fast on the day of the sweat, not to consume alcohol the day before, and not to wear any jewellery during the sweat. The men were asked to wear bathing trunks, and the women comfortable cotton gowns. Once we were seated in the lodge around the pit, hot rocks were brought in with a shovel and placed in the pit, and the lodge door was closed with heavy canvas tarps. There were thirteen of us crowded closely together. None of us had ever participated in a sweat before, and one of the female patients panicked when the lodge was closed and all was dark. She wanted to leave, but overcame her fear and stayed.

We had been told by Russell that if we found the sweat too hot or were in some way uncomfortable and wished to leave, we should simply say 'all my children' or 'all my relations,' which is the Cree way of asking for the door to be opened to allow someone to leave. But all the participants overcame their fears and endured the heat until the end. Fortunately, Russell did not make the sweat as hot as he would have for native patients. As usual, the sweat consisted of four rounds of praying, chanting to the rhythm of a rattle, and short talks by Russell, interspersed with the sprinkling of herbal water on the hot rocks to create medicated steam.

The experience was so satisfying to the patients, some of whose lesions virtually peeled off afterwards, that Russell agreed to come to Edmonton again and perform another one. Altogether there were three 'official' sweats for the patients, and an extra one to include spouses and children of both patients and researchers. Some patients reported having seen unusual lights during the sweat, and one woman excitedly described the experience of hearing the cry of the eagle.

The sweats were followed by eating fresh fruits and berries and dishes prepared by various patients. We drank natural fruit juices to replace the water lost through perspiration during the sweat.

Following the third sweat, the experiment was considered complete. A thanking ceremony took place at David Young's acreage. Each patient thanked Russell and presented him with a gift as a token of his or her gratitude. He reminded them that credit for the improvement in their psoriasis should be given to the Great Spirit, and since the Great Spirit was always around they could expect to see continued improvement.

A month later the patients met for the last time at the clinic so a physician could document their progress. Six patients were considered significantly improved. The other four, despite having shown earlier improvement, had reverted to their original conditions.

These results were less impressive than Russell had anticipated, and he was disappointed. Several times he offered explanations for why these non-native patients were healing more slowly than native patients. One suggestion was that 'they're not out in the fresh air much.' Another suggestion was that when

Russell came to Edmonton he treated patients for only a day, whereas when natives come to his house for treatment they get 'doctored for three solid days.' He also felt that different rates of improvement among patients might be related to the amount of praying they had done. The researchers pointed out that it was important to remember that Russell had run out of herbs early in the project, and that new roots had had to be collected in the winter when their chemical properties might be considerably altered. Also, because of the bad smell of the solution placed on the skin, it was felt that some of the patients may not have applied the medicine as regularly as they should have. In any case, Russell decided that in the future non-native patients who wished to be treated for psoriasis would have to come to the reserve and undergo the same three-day treatment as native patients. This has resulted in much more impressive results, including the case of Sandra, described in the previous chapter.

Russell's active involvement with the Psoriasis Research Project and his willingness to allow documentation of the sacred rituals involved is unusual and has caused some controversy within the native community and among health-care professionals. Within the native community there are some who support his endeavours and others who consider him to be disclosing sacred knowledge that should be kept within the native community. There is also the concern that the principles and values involved in traditional Indian medicine will be exposed once again to ridicule and exploitation. Some believe that if herbal combinations are revealed they will be used by drug companies for profit.

Criticism of the research project from within the Western medical system arises from lack of understanding of the context and scope of native therapy, which is considered to be outside the boundaries of modern, 'scientific' medicine. Near the completion of the research project we received a copy of a letter from the president of the Dermatological Association of Alberta to the University of Alberta medical school, questioning the use of university research funds for the study of such ostensibly unscientific activities. The unwillingness, indeed inability, of many doctors to recognize native medicine and therapy as a resource in a modern primary health-care system is not uncommon. In many ways this is a Catch-22 situation: because members of the medical profession do not extend recognition to treatments outside the scope of Western medicine, it is difficult to obtain the funding and research personnel needed to conduct scientific inquiry into the efficacy of native medicine.

Despite the controversy, Russell is continuing his efforts to prove that native medicine works. Although he is not willing to take part in any more experiments that attempt to 'control' the treatment environment, as was done to the best of our ability in the Psoriasis Research Project, he is open to new methods and arrangements, as the remaining two chapters illustrate.

❦ Two Case Histories

Early in 1987, Russell Willier phoned David Young from the Sucker Creek Reserve to ask a favour. 'I need a doctor who is willing to work with me,' he said. 'There are some things I can't do, mainly those things requiring surgery. It would also be very useful to have access to modern equipment, such as an x-ray machine, to check on how a patient is doing.'

Russell went on to explain that he had a female patient, Flora Cardinal, who had been diagnosed, at a clinic in Edmonton, as having cancer. According to Russell, Flora's cancer had been detected twenty-two years earlier, when she was sixteen years old, but it had gone into remission and she had given birth to several children. In 1986 she began to experience severe pains in her lower abdomen, so she went to a cancer clinic for tests. It was discovered that she had cancer of the cervix, and she was given numerous radiation and chemotherapy treatments, the longest one lasting for thirty-seven hours. Flora lost a lot of weight and her hair fell out, but on completion of the treatment the x-rays showed no signs of cancer.

After several months, however, Flora began to experience severe pains, her weight dropped, and she was having difficulty in urinating. She returned to the cancer clinic and described her symptoms. On the basis of these symptoms, but apparently without further lab tests, Flora was informed that the cancer had returned and had spread. It was assumed that tumours were putting pressure on her urethra, making it difficult for her to urinate. A plastic tube was inserted through her right side into her bladder so that urine could drain into a plastic bag attached to the end of the tube. Flora was notified that she was in a terminal stage, that nothing could be done for her, and that it would be best for her to return home and prepare to die. Doctors estimated she had approximately two weeks remaining.

Flora and her husband, Stu, went to see Russell as a last resort. After meditating on her problem, Russell said that he was not convinced Flora had cancer, and that he would put her on a herbal tea made from a combination of plants. After taking the tea for a couple of weeks, Flora, who had been extremely weak after returning home from the clinic, regained some strength and a little weight. Most important, she was still alive.

It was at this point that Russell telephoned me. He said that the herbal medicine had reduced the pain and swelling in the upper abdomen, and that Flora had regained the ability to urinate 'with her usual equipment.' He said, however, that Flora still had an infected area in the lower abdomen that was constantly discharging pus and fluid. Russell wanted to find a doctor who would be willing to scrape the uterus and thereby speed up the healing process. He also wanted the doctor to remove the plastic tube from her side, as he felt it was an unnecessary irritant.

I said I would try to find a medical doctor who might be willing to help him with such procedures. Over the next couple of weeks, I made inquiries among friends about a doctor who might be approached to help Russell. I remembered hearing about Dr Steven Aung, a Chinese MD and acupuncturist who runs a clinic in Edmonton and who was acquiring a considerable reputation for his knowledge of alternative therapies. I reached Dr Aung over the telephone and explained Russell's request. Dr Aung said he had heard about the Psoriasis Research Project. He expressed a keen interest in native medicine and said he would be happy to assist Russell in any way he could. I was pleased with this news and immediately telephoned Russell and explained that he should make an appointment for Flora with Dr Aung. I said that I would meet him and Flora at Dr Aung's office to introduce them to the doctor.

A meeting was arranged for 8 May 1987. Russell, Flora, Stu, Grant Ingram, and I arrived at the doctor's office. We were greeted by Dr Aung, who ushered us inside. After I had made the introductions, Dr Aung said he would like to write down Flora's history to date. He took notes while Stu went over past events. From time to time, Flora supplemented Stu's account with details of her own. We emphasized to Dr Aung that we hoped he would not pay undue attention to the official medical record from the cancer clinic but that he would start with a 'clean slate' and make his own independent evaluation of Flora's condition. Russell reiterated his desire to have the uterus scraped and the plastic tube removed. He also requested a blood transfusion for Flora, as she appeared to be anaemic.

After recording Flora's history, Dr Aung took her to another room and did a brief physical examination of her lower pelvic area. After they returned to the office, the doctor expressed the opinion that Flora's pain might be due not to cancer but to the build-up of scar tissue resulting from extended radiation treatment. He said that he would not know for certain until a complete physical examination could be done. He said that he was leaving soon on a trip to China and would not be able to conduct a complete physical until his return at the end of May. He ordered a series of lab tests for later that afternoon and asked us to come back a couple of days later to discuss the results.

When we met Dr Aung again at the clinic, he concurred with Russell's opinion that Flora was anaemic, but said that the lab tests had not revealed a low enough haemoglobin count to justify a blood transfusion. He prescribed iron pills instead. Flora soon discontinued taking the iron pills because she had an allergic reaction to them. Dr Aung also made arrangements for Flora to see another doctor, who was affiliated with one of the hospitals in Edmonton, while he was in China. He said he had worked with the doctor before and that she would be sympathetic to Flora's case. Flora and Stu were a little sceptical about seeing an 'orthodox' medical doctor again. They felt she would probably read the official medical history supplied by the cancer clinic and say the same things they had heard before: that it was a terminal case and that all that could be done was to try to ease the pain.

On 26 May, Lise, Grant, and I met Russell, Flora, and Stu at the palliative care unit of the hospital. The doctor was busy, so after the receptionist had recorded the necessary information, we all waited in the hall where we could hear cries of pain from terminal patients. Eventually, the doctor appeared. I was prepared to introduce Russell, who had made the long trip with Flora in order to hear what the doctor had to say, but the doctor asked for Flora and immediately whisked her away to a private office to go over the official medical record and conduct an examination. The doctor eventually reappeared and asked to talk to Stu. I intervened, to introduce Russell and myself, and explained that Russell would like to go over the case with her. She said she could give him about two minutes as she had to attend a meeting. Leaving Flora in the examination room, the doctor took Stu and Russell to another room.

Stu and Russell soon reappeared, without the doctor. They did not look happy. Stu explained that the doctor had informed them that Flora appeared to be experiencing some kind of re mission, but that they should not get their hopes up. The cancer would undoubtedly become active again, at which time it would probably be worse than ever. The doctor did not order further lab tests and refused to have the plastic tube removed or to authorize scraping the uterus, as such a procedure could cause bleeding that would be difficult to control. She also refused to authorize a blood transfusion but did give Flora a salve to be placed in the uterus to reduce infection. Stu said he would not inform Flora of the doctor's prognosis as he felt it would hurt her morale. He expressed anger that the interview had gone just as they had predicted, saying that they would never go to see another doctor again, except for Dr Aung, who, he felt, should be given another chance.

Russell said very little, but indicated that he didn't think any of them should come back again unless it was made very clear to Dr Aung that they wanted something quite different from him than they had received from other doctors. Russell said that it was very important to give Flora hope and to let her know that she would get well with the medicine he was giving her. The only reason for bringing medical doctors into the picture was to have the uterus scraped so the healing process would be speeded up. I promised to write a letter to Dr Aung explaining their concerns and to have it waiting for him on his return from China. When Flora rejoined us, Stu and Flora left for home. The trip home was very difficult for Flora as the salve that had been placed in her uterus caused considerable discomfort.

Two days after their return home, the doctor from the palliative care unit called Flora to say that she had reconsidered and would authorize the blood transfusion. She asked Stu and Flora to return to Edmonton. Because of the distance, Stu asked the doctor to arrange to have the transfusion done in the hospital at High Prairie. This was done, and Flora received four pints of blood. She reacted negatively to the transfusion, experiencing vomiting, diarrhoea, rapid weight loss, and depression, whereupon she resumed treatment with Russell. At this point, Russell changed his therapy. On the assumption that the plastic tube circumvented Flora's urinary system, thereby not allowing his medicine to reach where it should, Russell closed off the plastic tube for several hours at a time; during these intervals he administered a herbal medicine that caused Flora to eliminate small amounts of urine in the normal way. Russell also administered a herb that causes contractions and speeds up childbirth. Flora experienced pronounced contractions and said she felt the pain move downward to the pelvic area, where it seemed as though she were about to drop something. The pain continued to be severe. Although she tried different drugs previously prescribed by doctors to ease the pain, nothing seemed to help except Tylenol 3.

When Dr Aung returned, a new appointment was set up for 24 June 1987. We all met at Dr Aung's office. He made no mention of the letter but pledged that he would approach Flora's case with an open mind and would use diagnostic and treatment techniques based upon a much more holistic understanding of how the body functions than is the case with most MDs, who tend to be over-specialized in their training. Dr Aung then took Flora to another room for a physical examination. He invited Russell to attend the examination, but Russell declined because he felt Flora would be shy about having him there. Dr Aung and Flora returned in about twenty minutes. Dr Aung did not say much about the results of the physical examination, but said he was going to give Flora acupuncture and that we were welcome to watch.

We went to another room, where Flora lay down on an examination bench. Dr Aung had her hold a ground wire in one hand while he used an electromagnetic probe attached to a meter to measure Flora's Qi force through the different meridians, to which he gained access by touching points on the sides of her fingertips. As he touched a point, the meter would register a reading for the Qi level in the heart meridian, lung meridian, kidney meridian, genital-urinary meridian, and so on. He did this first on the right hand, where all the readings were lower than normal, and then on the left hand, where the readings were also below normal, but not as low as for the right side. On neither side was the reading for the kidney area as low as for the other meridians.

To provide a context for Flora's Qi, Dr Aung measured Russell's Qi level. The machine made a strange noise, and the meter swung to the right as far as it could go. 'Russell's Qi level is right off the screen,' Dr Aung said. He took Russell's hand to get a direct feel for his Qi, then said, 'He has so much Qi.' Turning to Russell, he said, 'you are also losing a lot of Qi. You need to learn some techniques for retaining it more effectively. If you can do that you will be a more powerful healer.' Dr Aung measured my Qi level and said that it was also high but that I was losing it even faster than Russell. Finally, he measured Grant and announced that he could hardly detect any Qi at all.

Dr Aung then gave Flora an acupuncture treatment. After thinking about which points to use, he would locate a point, push a plastic tube containing a disposable needle against the point, tap the end of the tube to insert the needle into the point, and withdraw the tube. He repeated this procedure a number of times, leaving needles at various points in Flora's feet, legs, abdomen, wrists, chest, and the top of her head. After all the needles were in place, he clipped wires to the needles and attached them to a voltage regulator, which fed current into each acupuncture point.

Dr Aung used additional wires to link the Qi channels together in specific combinations relevant to the therapy being done. The aims were to 'free' the flow of Qi at points where it was blocked and to balance the flow of Qi in the body. It is a 'tuning' process designed to help the body resist disease and do its own healing – Russell would say 'to trigger the body,' while Western doctors would say 'to stimulate the immune system.'

Electricity was allowed to flow through Flora's body for approximately fifteen minutes. She described the sensation as a 'tickle.' One needle, placed in her leg, was to reduce depression. Flora giggled during the treatment, and her husband Stu remarked that it was the first time he had seen Flora so happy in a long time. Another needle was inserted to stimulate the appetite. Flora remarked that she thought she could smell chicken noodle soup. When the needles were removed Flora said the pains in her abdomen were gone.

The next day Dr Aung arranged for Flora to have ultrasound tests to determine whether she had a tumour or abscess that might be causing the discharge from her vagina. Russell requested that anything removed from Flora be put in a bottle and given to him so he could add tobacco and seal the bottle to prevent the spirit of the disease from escaping and returning to Flora. Dr Aung said he had no trouble understanding that request, as there was a similar practice among indigenous healers in Burma, the country of his birth. Dr Aung asked us to come back to discuss the results of the tests.

Several days later when we met Dr Aung at his clinic, he informed us that the ultrasound tests were not completely successful. Flora had been requested to drink extra water to cause her abdominal tissues to swell, but because of the drainage tube inserted through her stomach, liquid did not reach the lower abdominal area, so the ultrasound tests could only be done for her stomach and the upper part of her abdomen. The tests did not reveal any tumours. Dr Aung said that the only way to know what was happening in the pelvic area would be to take a look. Because of the extreme sensitivity in that area, however, this procedure would have to wait. He did, however, take a tissue swab, the analysis of which did not indicate cancer. Dr Aung gave Flora a second acupuncture treatment to control pain in the abdomen. Flora and Stu then returned home.

Flora Cardinal died at the end of 1988, nearly two years after beginning treatment with Russell.

Her death leaves unanswered questions. When Flora returned to the cancer clinic, had the cancer returned and spread, or was she incorrectly diagnosed? If the cancer had returned, Russell's herbal medicine may be responsible for keeping her alive for nearly two years despite the fact that she was given two weeks to live. Was Flora's pain due to scar tissue caused by radiation treatment? If so, Russell's medicine greatly reduced the extent of scarring, since tests did not reveal abnormal tissue in the upper abdomen, and the pain was confined to the pelvic area. In either case, Russell's therapy appears to have been beneficial.

Regardless of how these questions are answered, Flora's case has led to co-operation between Russell Willier and Dr Aung. Dr Aung refers selected patients to Russell, and Russell refers native patients to Dr Aung when the assistance of modern diagnostic and treatment procedures is needed. Dr Aung administers acupuncture to control pain and to balance the flow of energy in the body. Russell administers the herbal medications. Native patients treated by Russell and Dr Aung receive the best of both the traditional and modern worlds of medicine.

Dr Aung has become involved with psoriasis patients seeking help from Russell, authorizing the use of hospital photographic services and recording the progress of patients. When a sufficient number of cases have been documented, Dr Aung, Russell, and

David plan to prepare articles for medical journals. We hope that this innovative experiment in cross-cultural medicine will help us develop a model that may eventually result in more interaction between native healers and medical doctors, with a consequent improvement in health care for natives and non-natives alike.

MICHIKO YOUNG

On 21 March 1987, Michiko Young, wife of David Young, came down with a high fever and diarrhoea. David Young's account of her illness follows.

Michiko stayed in bed, taking Tylenol to keep her temperature down. On the second day of her illness Michiko had a dream about going on a herb-collecting expedition with Russell: as Russell collected the herbs, Michiko took notes.

Since she showed no signs of improvement, I took Michiko to a clinic in a nearby town. The doctor diagnosed her condition as the flu. She was advised to stay in bed, drink plenty of liquids, and continue taking Tylenol to keep the fever down. After a few days, Michiko became very weak and was unable to sleep at night. On the third night after the visit to the clinic her nose began to bleed. We tried ice packs and pressure but were unable to stop the bleeding. We called the emergency room of the nearby hospital and tried the pressure method described to us over the telephone. When this did not work, we went to the emergency room at three in the morning. The nurse was unable to stop the bleeding and called the doctor. He was unable to come, as he was due in surgery. The nurse thoroughly cleared the nasal cavities of blood clots and reapplied pressure. The bleeding stopped eventually, Michiko's temperature returned to normal, and she was sent home.

As soon as she returned home, however, Michiko's temperature climbed to 105 degrees. She continued to weaken, so on 27 March I took her back to the doctor at the clinic. The doctor saw immediately that Michiko could hardly walk and was severely dehydrated, so she ordered a variety of tests, including chest x-rays. Michiko was admitted to the hospital.

The next day, Michiko was put on intravenous feeding and antibiotics, but she continued to deteriorate. She was transferred by ambulance to the university hospital in Edmonton, and I was informed over the telephone that I should meet her there. When our son and I arrived at the emergency room, Michiko was barely conscious and did not recognize either of us. We kept asking her how she felt, but she could only reply that she was tired. She was examined by a doctor, admitted to the hospital, and put in a room with another woman. The following day she was transferred to a private room in the intensive care unit and placed in isolation because of the fear of contagious disease. Michiko was extremely dehydrated by this time, because her fever had not dropped substantially in ten days. The nurses set up a fan to blow over a block of ice in an attempt to bring down the temperature, but to little avail.

As Michiko continued to get worse, the doctors decided to take her off antibiotics and switch to another type of medication. Unable to reach a diagnosis, they ordered blood tests to be taken every half-hour. On 31 March I was informed that the doctors could not isolate the cause, but that it appeared to be something similar to Legionnaire's Disease. They were hopeful that the fever could be brought down, but they were concerned that Michiko was so dehydrated she might not be able to survive.

That evening, thoroughly discouraged with modern medicine, I called Russell and asked for his help. Russell said that he'd had a vision instructing him to collect a particular set of herbs, as someone would be calling. He said the herbs were ready and that he would be at my house early the next morning to make preparations for treatment.

As soon as Russell arrived we began ritual preparations. The first step was to light a piece of dried fungus collected from an old willow tree and purify the house. While I took the smoking fungus in a clockwise direction around every room of the house, Russell left a strand of woven sweetgrass in the dining-room for

Michiko to burn when she returned home. Although Michiko was near death, leaving the sweetgrass was a sign of confidence in the power of the Great Spirit and his helpers.

While a pan of water was being boiled, Russell and our son, Chris, sat at the dining-room table cutting up several different kinds of herbs. When the water was ready the herbs were added. Four small branches from four different kinds of trees, representing the four cardinal directions, were added, one at a time, and leaned against the top edge of the pan in the direction each branch represented. The resulting herbal tea was placed in two glass jugs for transport to the hospital.

Then we performed the pipe ceremony. Russell lighted a ceremonial, stone-bowled pipe and passed it to Chris and me, again in a clockwise direction. He said it was important to see the fire through the stone; if we could not it would mean that Michiko would not survive. Russell said that the spirits had revealed to him that it was a tight situation, and he wasn't sure whether we were in time. Russell said he could see the fire through the stone bowl of the pipe, but I could not see it. So Russell told me to take the pipe into the bathroom where it was completely dark and see if I could see the flame. I did so, but still wasn't sure I saw anything. I brought the pipe back to the dining-room and it was passed around three or four more times. Russell then announced that the spirit helpers were already on the way to the hospital and would begin helping Michiko before we got there.

We arrived at the hospital just before noon. Michiko was in isolation. I told the nurse who I was, and she wanted to know who Russell was so I said he was a relative. On the way to the hospital we had debated about whether to tell the hospital staff that Russell intended to treat Michiko. We decided to conceal the purpose of his visit, believing that the hospital might give him permission to burn sweetgrass in the room but not to administer medicine to Michiko.

Within a few minutes, the doctor in charge had called in several specialists and we met in a conference room. The doctors expressed their opinions about what kind of infection Michiko might have, but nobody knew for sure. They said that they had administered different drugs intravenously but that none of them seemed to help. They currently had her on a massive dose of a drug that was used to combat mycoplasm, their best guess of what she might have. They were going to take a spinal tap to see if she had spinal meningitis and whether it had moved to her brain. They suspected that it had, as Michiko, who is an accountant, was unable to answer such simple questions as 'What is the sum of two plus two?' They expressed the opinion that if the fever had gone to her brain Michiko would have little chance of recovery.

We were allowed to see Michiko after donning white gowns and masks. When we entered the room Michiko opened her eyes. She apparently recognized Russell, as her eyes lit up and she said, 'My doctor is here.'

'She looks terrible,' Russell said, looking at the intravenous equipment and oxygen mask. 'I want all that stuff off of her first thing. Then I can treat her.' I had been dreading this moment.

'I don't think we should have it taken off,' I said. 'Michiko is so weak that the oxygen and intravenous feeding may be all that is keeping her alive. If we take it off, she may not live long enough to respond to your herbal doctoring.'

Russell thought for a minute and then said, 'Well, okay. In most cases I would insist that it be done my way or not at all, but I'll compromise this time. We'll leave the equipment on and begin herbal treatment right away.'

The first thing Russell did was chew up a piece of sweet-smelling root, which he blew on Michiko's face and rubbed on her forehead. The fragrance filled the room. Then Russell said, 'Let's get her to drink the tea.' We poured tea into a glass and persuaded Michiko to drink a little through a straw. The nurse came back into the room, saw the tea, and said, 'Where did that stuff come from?' She dumped the tea in the bathroom sink. As soon as she left we refilled the glass and gave Michiko some more. Michiko was able to drink nearly half a glass at a time before the nurse would come back into the room and dump out the tea. Another nurse, however, did not dump out the tea, but simply said, 'You've been giving her some extra stuff, haven't you?' I didn't reply, and she let it pass.

Russell and I took turns staying in the room, giving Michiko the tea whenever we had the chance. Russell said that the important thing was to get as much tea into her as possible and not to let her drink the ice-water that the nurses kept bringing into the room. Ice-water was the worst thing she could take, he believed. Michiko drank about three glasses of herb tea over the next four hours.

At four in the afternoon the doctor in charge informed us that the fever had not gone to Michiko's brain. 'Don't get your hopes up yet,' the doctor said, 'but your wife seems to be doing better. Her fever is coming down and her blood pressure is up.'

'Did you notice any particular time that she started to improve?' I asked. The doctor gave me a funny look and said, 'Well, her vital signs started improving about two o'clock.' Russell and I looked at each other.

That evening, Russell and I had been invited to dinner at the home of a colleague in my department. As we were about to leave, I told Russell about Michiko's diarrhoea and that the doctors had not been able to stop it ever since she had been admitted into the hospital. 'Why didn't you tell me this when you telephoned?' he said. 'I could have brought something along. Never mind. Maybe we can collect something on the way to your friend's house.' As we were driving to my friend's place, we passed a wooded area along the river. 'Stop.' Russell said. 'I don't have my knife along, but I can use my teeth to collect a little bark from a special kind of tree.' He went into the woods and soon returned with a piece of green bark. 'This should do the trick,' Russell said. 'We shouldn't stay too long for dinner because we have to be back to treat Michiko before the sun sets, or she can still die.'

When we arrived at my friend's house, dinner was ready and we sat down and had a good meal. When we were finished Russell said, 'Well, we'd better get going.' My friend and his wife were surprised that we were leaving so early. 'We have to be back before the sun sets,' Russell told our puzzled hosts. We jumped up from the table, said a quick goodbye, and climbed into the car just as the sun was beginning to set. 'We'd better hurry,' Russell said. 'It's going to be close.' I broke the speed limit getting to the hospital, about fifteen minutes away. We parked the car and ran for the hospital just as the sun went out of sight. Fortunately, the elevator was waiting. We dashed out of the elevator on the fifth floor and ran down the hall past the startled nurses. We went into Michiko's room and looked out the window. We were able to see the top of the sun as it was disappearing over the horizon. 'We're okay,' said Russell, who had been chewing the bark. He took the bark from his mouth and placed it in Michiko's mouth and got her to swallow it along with some herbal tea. She made a face because of the bitterness.

I was relieved that we had made it in time. Michiko's diarrhoea stopped immediately, to the surprise of the nurses. The following day a slight case of diarrhoea returned, so Russell gave her another piece of bark and asked her to chew it up herself. The diarrhoea did not return.

Russell stayed in Edmonton for three days, taking care of personal business and checking on Michiko. I returned home in the evenings but spent most of the day sitting in Michiko's hospital room, making sure that she continued to drink the herbal tea. Russell announced that he had to go home, but that he would return in a couple of days with a root that would restore Michiko's appetite. Michiko kept saying that she was not hungry and that everything tasted terrible. The only thing she would take was the herbal tea.

Two days later Russell returned with a bag of roots and instructed me to make tea. I did so, and went to the hospital with three jugs of tea. The nurses gave me suspicious looks, but didn't say anything. Russell warned me not to give Michiko more than one glass of the appetite stimulant or it would cause her to gain too much weight. I found this hard to believe, as Michiko was thin even before her illness.

The next day Michiko sat up in bed and allowed me to spoon-feed her. She preferred Jello, canned fruit, and other easily digestible foods. Gradually, over the next few days, she began eating more and more, saying that she was constantly hungry. This was when we knew that she was going to be all right. We were told we no longer needed the gowns and masks, and other visitors were permitted. The doctors acknowledged that Michiko was improving and expressed surprise at the speed of her recovery.

Michiko's mental faculties remained impaired. She had no idea of what the date was, could not perform simple math problems, and was not able to write in a straight line. The doctors felt that the high fever over such a long period of time might have caused brain damage. They said that it was also possible the massive doses of drugs were causing her to be drowsy and unable to respond in a normal manner.

Michiko began to spend some time each day sitting up in bed, but she continued to be fed intravenously and to wear an oxygen mask. Occasionally, I was allowed to wheel her out to sit in the sun. She tired easily, however, and would soon ask to go back to her room so she could sleep. The nurses encouraged her to get up to use the bathroom. This proved to be quite a task, as the oxygen had to be unplugged from the wall and plugged into a portable tank, and the intravenous unit had to be dragged along. The nurses began to experience great difficulty in keeping the intravenous needle in Michiko's arm, as the major veins had collapsed and her arms were black and blue from the numerous needle insertions. Michiko asked for the intravenous feeding to be stopped. This request was rejected, as the doctors wanted her to stay on the intravenous medication. They said that an oral medication was available, but that it tended to cause stomach problems.

Keeping the needle in Michiko's arm proved to be nearly impossible, so the intravenous equipment was removed. Oxygen was continued, because Michiko felt too tired without it.

Michiko stayed in the hospital for three weeks. During that time, various specialists came to see her. Tests continued to be done, and her vital signs were monitored regularly. We were never able to get any answers about the cause of her illness. It was difficult to know whom to talk to, since Michiko was being seen by so many doctors. Although each team of specialists would record something in the log-book at the nurses' station, no one doctor seemed to know the whole picture.

The most useful explanation I received was from the brother of the colleague whose dinner Russell, Chris, and I had left so suddenly. The brother, a medical doctor, was visiting from Detroit and happened to meet me in the parking lot at the university. He said he had heard about my wife's problem and went on to say that it sounded as though Michiko's illness was a yeast-based infection. He explained that our bodies contain various kinds of yeasts (such as *Candida albicans*). These yeasts are normally kept in check by bacteria that also live in the body. When Michiko had first been admitted to the local hospital, the doctors assumed she had a bacteria-based infection and gave her antibiotics. But these succeeded only in killing off the bacteria that keep the yeasts in check. Thus, Michiko deteriorated quickly. Although they changed the medication when Michiko was transferred to the university hospital, drugs to combat yeasts and viruses are not nearly as well developed as drugs to combat bacteria. Therefore, he hypothesized, it proved to be very difficult to bring down Michiko's fever, especially when she was in such a weakened condition.

Michiko was discharged from the hospital on 16 April. She was relieved to be home, since it meant she could finally get some decent sleep without being awakened every half-hour for tests. She convalesced at home for another month, finally returning to work approximately two and a half months after she had fallen ill. But her troubles were not over. Within a few weeks her hair started coming out in clumps, and before long she was nearly bald. We bought a wig so she could continue work without embarrassment. She also applied bear grease that Russell had given her and began taking large doses of vitamins, particularly B, E, and lecithin. Her hair then stopped falling out and started to grow again.

Michiko regained full health. Would she have died without help from Russell's medicine and his spirit helpers? It is impossible to prove one way or another, but in our minds we are convinced that Russell made a significant difference. He was able to inspire confidence in both Michiko and myself in a way that the doctors and nurses at the hospital could not. The herbal treatments appeared to have been effective. Michiko's fever went down within two hours after drinking the herbal tea. Her diarrhoea stopped shortly after swallowing the bark, and she started eating within a day after taking the herbal appetite stimulant. Are these coincidences? We do not think so. The doctors, of course, who did not even know Michiko was being treated by a medicine man, would naturally attribute the results to the fact that the modern drugs eventually took effect. I am sure they would be less eager to claim responsibility for not recognizing the seriousness of Michiko's condition sooner or for the fact that initially she was given medication that nearly proved fatal. They would probably be a little chagrined to know that a simple piece of bark stopped Michiko's diarrhoea, a condition that had significantly contributed to her dehydration for more than a week and that had failed to respond to modern drugs.

When it was all over, I asked Russell if he felt it had been wise to compromise with me and leave Michiko in the care of the doctors when he had wanted to discontinue intravenous feeding, medication, and oxygen. He thought for a moment, then said, 'I think it was the right choice. Michiko might not have survived without the oxygen and intravenous feeding. In fact, I am more convinced than ever that I should be working with doctors. Even though my medicine is better – at least for certain problems – the doctors have equipment that is very useful. We should be able to help each other out rather than having to sneak me into the hospital.'

We cannot help but wonder if the day will come when physicians will realize that two dozen specialists may not be as effective as one caring family doctor and that modern drug therapy can produce as many problems as solutions. It may be an exaggeration to say that a hospital is no place for sick people, but I feel that modern medicine almost cost me my wife's life. If another disease cripples me or a member of my family, I will not necessarily refuse the help of a hospital; but you can be sure that I will bring in the help of a traditional healer like Russell Willier much earlier.

❦ Creative Encounters

Russell Willier and the authors of this book have been changed as a result of the cross-cultural encounters we have had with each other over the past five years. Before becoming involved in joint research with anthropologists, Russell was relatively unknown, except to native people in the Sucker Creek area and to a scattering of patients in Edmonton. The Psoriasis Research Project and the dissemination of its results in videotapes, journals, books, international conferences, and the media have made Russell known to many people around the world. This growing reputation has reinforced Russell's belief that he has been 'called' to lead a revitalization movement, a movement that will bring new life to native culture and values, not by retreating into the past and attempting to restore pristine independence, but by making the strengths of native culture known to the outside world. If this can be done, it will demonstrate the universal applicability of native religion and medicine and stimulate a sense of pride on the part of native young people.

The focal point for the revitalization movement is to be a healing centre on the reserve – a centre that is to be open to both native and non-native people. The goal of the centre is to promote native culture, with an emphasis on native religion and medicine. It is to be a co-operative endeavour between Russell and other interested medicine men.

Russell is proceeding with plans to develop the healing centre at what he perceives to be considerable risk to himself and his family. Such a centre would not only break with tradition but would arouse jealousy. Therefore, he has decided to proceed slowly, hoping in the meantime to attain the shaking tipi. If he had the shaking tipi, no one could touch him. He would have the power to neutralize or return curses, send and receive messages, read thoughts 'from one ocean to the other,' and see the future. He would have almost unlimited power as long as he followed the right road. He could then proceed with the healing centre without fear for the safety of himself or his family.

The first step in planning the healing centre has been to set up a non-profit organization known as the Traditional Native Healing Society. The organization's objectives are to: (1) promote, encourage, and teach Indian culture, customs, and values; (2) provide for the treatment and prevention of diseases and ailments, incorporating traditional Indian remedies and practices; (3) experiment with adapting traditional healing practices and remedies to the modern situation in terms of professional services and facilities for patients and families.

Russell considers the educational aspect of the centre to be just as important as its healing function. He feels that it is critical to educate young people about the dangers of alcohol and drug abuse before it's too late. He emphasizes that 'it's much better to prevent problems than to have to deal with them after the damage has been done.'

Recently, the Traditional Native Healing Society was granted charitable status by the federal government. This was a big step forward, as it implies recognition on the part of the government that native medicine has value. It also means that individuals and corporations can now make tax-deductible contributions to the society. Russell hopes that the publicity stemming from the Psoriasis Research Project will encourage people 'from all over' to donate money to help build the physical facilities necessary to accommodate the hundreds of people who are already seeking help. Until the facilities are in place, there is very little Russell can do for outsiders, as treating people intensively over several days requires a place for them to sleep and eat, at a minimum.

It has proved unworkable to try to handle patients in his home, because it places too great a burden on his family and personal life.

The non-profit organization has a board of directors consisting of Russell and influential people from both the native and non-native communities. Russell realizes that it would be advantageous to set up the healing centre as a band project. Such an arrangement would make it easier to meet government regulations and obtain government assistance. He insists, however, that he will never allow this to happen, as it would only mean trouble in the future. Band projects are carried on at the whim of the band council, whose membership changes frequently. The original board of directors might work hard to achieve the goals of the organization, but directors appointed later might use the project as a way of lining their own pockets. Although the band will not be involved formally in the project, it has provided Russell with written approval for the project.

The same principle holds in relation to investors. The healing centre could be set up as a private company with dividend-paying shares. But there is insufficient investment money on the reserve, and investors would most likely be wealthy Indian bands or non-native interests from the city. In either case, it would mean outside control. A non-profit organization appears to be the best way to raise money without losing control.

Russell has decided to 'start small' by buying used mobile homes to be set up on a vacant area of land near his house on the reserve. The mobile homes will provide sleeping and cooking facilities for patients, space for a receptionist to take telephone calls and help patients arrange visits to the reserve, and a place for storing herbs and treating patients. There will also be three sweat-lodges, each run by a medicine man (or woman) with a particular specialty, such as contagious diseases, chronic conditions, or psychological counselling.

The healing centre will provide a bridge between native and non-native culture. Treatment will be traditional, consisting of 'sweats' and the administration of herbal medicines. Patients will be interviewed by native doctors, assigned to individual quarters, and served food to which they are accustomed. This arrangement will ensure privacy for both the patients and the Willier family. In line with native tradition, there will be no set fee schedule. Prospective patients, however, will be asked to make a minimum donation to the non-profit organization, regardless of the treatment or the benefits gained. They will also be charged a daily rate for food and accommodation. Donations and grants will be sought from other sources to help support the activities of the healing centre once it is in operation.

Yvonne thinks that the healing centre has little chance of materializing. She feels that Russell is a dreamer who has neither the temperament nor the experience to make a healing centre a viable enterprise. Her outspoken doubts about the project are a source of friction. Russell feels that a good Indian wife should be supportive of his plans. Moreover, he would like Yvonne to be the bookkeeper for the healing centre and to help write children's books about native culture and values that will be used in educational programs associated with the centre. Yvonne has good business sense and would be able to handle the financial records and fill out the many forms connected with a business operation. Yvonne, however, has a career of her own. She is an experienced seamstress who makes an equal contribution to the family budget by taking orders for parkas, moccasins, and traditional arts and crafts. She also teaches courses at the vocational training school in nearby Grouard. Yvonne enjoys sewing and teaching and is determined not to give up her own career in order to keep the books for a project she feels has little chance of succeeding.

It was remarked earlier that Russell Willier's life was changed by the Psoriasis Research Project. In line with the objectives of this book, we must consider our role as anthropologists in this change. Has our role been constructive or not?

There is a growing literature on the history of the social sciences indicating that in the past anthropologists served the goals of colonialism and Western cultural imperialism. They may not have done this intentionally, but they did so nonetheless. Along with explorers and missionaries, anthropologists frequently paved the way for the businesses, military forces, and colonial governments that were to follow. They did so by making contact with isolated groups of people and by documenting local customs and values. These ethnographic descriptions were frequently of great use to colonial governments that desired to rule with a minimum of force and cost. Anthropologists have continued to be co-opted through the years for a variety of economic and political programs. This is not to cast aspersions upon the quality of the data gathered and the books written. Nevertheless, anthropologists are viewed with suspicion in many parts of the world because of their perceived close connection with the values and goals of the societies from which they come.

Suspicion of anthropologists seems fairly common among the native peoples of North America. Anthropologists have been perceived as researchers who come in for a brief time, get their data, and exploit that data for the rest of their lives, with very little long-term benefit to those who supplied the information.

We must ask, then, if this has been true of our relationship with Russell Willier. It cannot be denied that our work with him has promoted our own careers in that it has allowed us to write both this book and a variety of other materials. It could also be argued that the publicity we have generated has encouraged a relatively obscure native healer to strive for unrealistic goals and to pursue a path that will eventually lead to failure and disillusionment. In the words of Russell's wife, Yvonne, there is a danger that success has 'gone to his head' and that his plans may result in misery for the Willier family. Even worse, there is a belief among members of Russell's extended family that his ambition has entailed a 'price,' that price being the deaths of several close relatives over the past few years as a result of curses sent by individuals upset with Russell's innovations or jealous of his success. Although there have never been direct accusations, there is some indication that these deaths are attributed indirectly to our involvement with Russell.

These are serious matters, and considering them has at times caused us to believe that it might be best to discontinue research with Russell. There is another side to the story that must be considered, however. As we related earlier, Russell had a vision that he interpreted to mean that he had been selected to lead a revitalization movement. This feeling of having been chosen for a special mission is reinforced by incidents from his childhood.

Russell was perceived by his family to be an unusual boy because of his habit of rising early in the summer, around four or five in the morning, to go outside and observe the birds awakening and the flowers opening. Once, as a teenager, Russell was on a hunt with his father and uncle. The hunt was unsuccessful, and the uncle and father returned home empty-handed. Russell had a vision in which he saw two moose and their hiding place in the forest, and he returned home to tell the other hunters, but they did not believe him. Finally, an uncle consented to have a look. To his surprise, he and Russell found the moose where Russell had said they would be. The moose were shot, and Russell returned home again to secure additional assistance for butchering and carrying the moose out of the bush.

As a result of such experiences, Russell came to believe that he has a special purpose in life. But having lived a traditional life on the reserve, he felt trapped in a rather predictable lifestyle until the anthropologists came along. After getting to know David Young, Grant Ingram, and Lise Swartz, Russell became convinced that they fitted into the general scheme of things and would provide opportunities for him to realize his goals. In Russell's words, 'If you hadn't come along, someone else would have.' In a similar vein, Russell sometimes urged us to complete this book more rapidly. On one occasion he said, 'If you don't get this into print pretty soon, I'll give the story to someone else.'

It is not a simple matter of one-sided exploitation. Both sides have benefited from the relationship. If, at any time, Russell perceives that the relationship is having an adverse impact upon his progress, he will undoubtedly take steps to terminate the flow of information – though not necessarily the friendship that has developed over the years.

Our influence has extended beyond providing Russell with a

window on the world – a window that has allowed him to see new possibilities in the larger world of the 'white man' while at the same time allowing the rest of the world to see him. We have influenced his values and his decisions in numerous ways. When Russell and his brother were debating how to set up a structure for the clinic, we advised them to establish a non-profit organization instead of a private company. This advice was heeded and, at Russell's request, we found a lawyer at the University of Alberta who did the legal work free of charge. Although we have not hesitated to offer advice about such matters, we have placed limits on the nature of our involvement. Russell initially asked David Young to be on the board of directors for the healing centre. This offer was politely refused on the grounds that membership on the board of directors would constitute conflict of interest. David felt he could not continue to observe and document Russell's activities with sufficient objectivity if he were intimately involved in the official decision-making processes of the centre. Russell readily understood this point and never raised the issue again.

Russell has continued to ask for informal advice and help, however. He recently asked us to try to save the area of the Swan Hills that he and another medicine man hope to use for the instruction of young people in the summer. The area is in danger of being logged and is frequently invaded by snowmobilers. It would be no good for teaching survival skills or for vision-quest sites if it were stripped of trees or overrun by recreation enthusiasts. Russell claims that this area has been used for many generations for vision-quest purposes.

Russell and David Young made a trip to the relevant agencies to obtain maps. Armed with these, David is attempting to persuade the government to help preserve a portion of the Swan Hills for traditional native activities. If we cannot obtain government help, we may have to wage a media campaign and hope for public support. Such activities fall in the area of what is aptly called 'action anthropology,' a new orientation that entails advocacy of the rights of minority groups living within the confines of modern, pluralistic societies. Action anthropology is legitimate as long as the action is in response to requests coming from indigenous peoples themselves. Responding to such requests, if they accord with the anthropologists' own sense of social justice, is one of the few ways we have of helping the people on whom we rely for our research careers.

As the relationship with Russell Willier has grown over the years, it has gone beyond the simple exchange of ethnographic information to include assistance in dealing with 'white man's institutions.' When Russell came to the hospital in Edmonton to treat David Young's wife, as was described in the previous chapter, he stayed at the hospital for three days in the guise of a concerned relative, giving Michiko herbal medicine whenever the nurses left the room. As a consequence, David Young is more indebted to the healer than social scientists normally are to informants.

More recently, the Youngs' sixteen-year-old son, Chris, an adopted boy of native background, was not doing well in high school and had dropped out. When the problem was mentioned to Yvonne and Russell, they offered to have Chris live at their house for a while, so he could attend school in a nearby town and apprentice as a healer. Chris approved of this arrangement, as he had come to respect Russell and Yvonne over the years and had learned to identify with native culture. As a result of living with the Williers, Chris appears to have gained a new sense of purpose.

Like the warp and woof in woven fabric, the lives of social scientists and the people with whom they work can become intertwined in numerous ways and at different levels. At this point it would be absurd to claim that our study of Russell Willier and the development of his revitalization movement is objective or unbiased. But then, no ethnography is objective or unbiased. An ethnography is simply the author's description of an encounter between himself or herself and the person or people studied. Just as the 'natural' activities of subatomic particles cannot be observed directly because the amount of light necessary to allow such observation distorts the behaviour of the particles, so the anthropologist's study of any culture creates a new situation. We can only record encounters in which we are involved.

To return to Russell. He cannot go back to the simpler days before he met us. He continues to dream about his healing centre and about being able to make a living as a full-time medicine man. Despite the sizable obstacles in his path, he believes it is inevitable that he will find a way to bring his plans to fruition. While working to develop the healing centre, Russell continues to make a living as best he can. He treats a slow but steady stream of patients, guides big-game hunters from the United States, manages the band's buffalo herd, and does odd jobs around the reserve. Like his spirit helper the eagle, Russell tries to take a long-range view. He knows that his time will come.

❧ Select Bibliography

Bateson, G., and M.C. Bateson. 1987. *Angels Fear: Towards an Epistemology of the Sacred*. New York: Macmillan

Capra, F. 1984. *The Tao of Physics*. New York: Bantam Books

Cardinal, H. 1977. *The Rebirth of Canada's Indians*. Edmonton: Hurtig

Clifford, J., and M. Marcus, eds. 1986. *Writing Culture*. Berkeley: University of California Press

Eisenberg, D., and T.L. Wright. 1987. *Encounters with Qi: Exploring Chinese Medicine*. New York: Penguin Books

Gadamer, H. 1975. *Truth and Method*. London: Sheed and Ward

Ingram, G. 1989. 'An Insider's View of the Woods Cree Cursing System: An Anthropological Analysis.' MA diss., University of Alberta, Edmonton

Kaptchuk, O.M.D. 1983. *The Web That Has No Weaver: Understanding Chinese Medicine*. New York: Congdon and Weed

Martin, C. 1978. *Keepers of the Game: Indian-Animal Relationships and the Fur Trade*. Berkeley: University of California Press

O'Neil, J.D. 1986. 'The Politics of Health in the Fourth World: A Northern Canadian Example.' *Human Organization* 45 (2): 253–4

Swartz, L. 1987. 'A Cree Healer in Role Transition.' MA diss., University of Alberta, Edmonton

Swartz, L. 1988. 'Healing Properties of the Sweatlodge Ceremony.' In *Health Care Issues in the Canadian North*, ed. D.E. Young. Edmonton: Boreal Institute for Northern Studies

Tedlock. D. 1983. *The Spoken Word and the Work of Interpretation*. Philadelphia: University of Pennsylvania Press

Wallace, A.F.C. 1970. *Culture and Personality*. New York: Random Press

Watson, L.C., and M. Watson-Franke. 1985. *Interpreting Life Histories: An Anthropological Inquiry*. New Brunswick, NJ: Rutgers University Press

Young, D.E., ed. 1988. *Health Care Issues in the Canadian North*. Edmonton: Boreal Institute for Northern Studies

Young, D.E., G. Ingram, and L. Swartz. 1988. 'The Persistence of Traditional Medicine in the Modern World.' *Cultural Survival Quarterly* 12 (1): 38–41

Young, D.E., J. Morse, and R. McConnell. 1988. 'Documenting the Practice of a Traditional Healer: Methodological Problems and Issues.' In *Health Care Issues in the Canadian North*, ed. D.E. Young, 89–94. Edmonton: Boreal Institute for Northern Studies

Young, D.E., J. Morse, L. Swartz, and G. Ingram. 1988. 'The Psoriasis Research Project: An Overview.' In *Health Care Issues in the Canadian North*, ed. D.E. Young, 76–87. Edmonton: Boreal Institute for Northern Studies

Young, D.E., J. Morse, L. Swartz, and R. McConnell. 1988. 'A Cree Indian Treatment for Psoriasis: A Longitudinal Study.' *Culture* 7 (2): 31–41

Young, D.E., and L. Swartz. 1985. *A Cree Healer*. Videotape. Edmonton: University of Alberta, Department of Radio and Television

– 1985. *The Psoriasis Research Project*. Videotape. Edmonton: University of Alberta, Department of Radio and Television

Young, D.E., and D. Wolf. 1983. 'The Adaptive Significance of Intracultural Diversity.' *Culture* 3 (2): 59–71

Zuk, D.R. 1988. 'The Native Medicine Man in Canada: An Annotated Bibliography.' MA diss., University of Alberta, Edmonton

❦ Index